MW00966126

The Ping Pong Diet

A Twenty-One Point

Plan for Sustainable Weight Loss

Dr. Chris Ko, M.D.

Copyright © 2014 Authored by Chris Ko
All rights reserved.

ISBN: 1500477532
ISBN 13: 978-1500477530

Table of Contents:

Note from the Author

This book is intended to supplement, not replace the advice of a trained health professional. You should consult your physician before engaging in any weight management. The ideas and information presented should be used in combination with the guidance and care of your physician. Weight loss has been associated with the development of kidney stones and gallstones. The author and publisher specifically disclaim any liability, loss, or risk personal or otherwise, incurred as a consequence, directly or indirectly, of the use and application of any of the contents of this book.

Introduction

"The doctor of the future will give no medicine, but will interest his patients in the care of the human frame, in diet, and in the cause and prevention of disease."

–Thomas Edison

Eat less and exercise more. It seems like the logical and simple strategy for weight loss. But if it is so simple, why are two-thirds of Americans still struggling with being overweight or obese? When conventional methods for treating a problem fail, it is time to look at the problem in an unconventional way.

Throughout this book, I will challenge the way you think about food and your body. You will learn that weight gain is not a simple matter of overconsumption; it's overconsumption of the *wrong* stuff. Rather than count calories, I will teach you to make the *quality* of your calories count. I will dispel the myth that exercise is an effective strategy for weight loss and promote the power of plants and protein. I will expose secrets that the processed food industry desperately want to keep hidden from you, while teaching you strategies that have helped others maintain significant weight loss.

I have drawn these strategies from medical studies as well as from my own clinical experience as an internist practicing weight management. Taken together, the knowledge I give you will not only help you successfully manage your weight, but also lead to meaningful change in your life and your health. And while my strategy is backed by science, effective weight management depends upon more than just empirical studies. Effective weight management is also more than a number on a scale and much more than the sum of the calories eaten.

Effective weight management is as much about the human spirit as it is about the human body. In order to truly inspire great change, you need to learn about the psychology of the human mind, and understand what drives behavior. Despite all my medical training, I credit an entirely different kind of training for helping me understand the power of the human spirit—my training in ping pong. That training took me to the small town of Lawrence, Kansas, during the summer of 1988.

Chapter 1: Go for the Gold!

"We will now be starting the championship match for the boys ten and under age group!" boomed the announcer. His voice echoed in the microphone and filled the gymnasium.

"The Junior Olympic finals match will be played between Eugene Huffington and Chris Ko!"

My heart quickened. All that time spent training in my parents' basement, practicing with the green ball machine monster, and the hours of sage advice from my coach had converged and brought me to this moment. I steeled myself, took a single deep breath, then walked out onto the gymnasium floor.

The bleachers were filled with spectators brimming with anticipation and excitement. This was an unusually large crowd for an event featuring the youngest age category. And the reason for this was the boy standing across the table from me—Eugene Huffington.

Eugene had a thin frame, pale skin, and shaggy red hair. But behind a seemingly frail exterior, lurked a boy with a fierce competitiveness and an attitude to match.

Eugene had become infamous in the table tennis community not just because he showed impressive talent at a young age, but because he exhibited a precocious flair for the dramatic. Think miniature John McEnroe, except Eugene threw his racquet onto a *table* tennis court. This was the Junior Olympics. We were kids. We all had our share of emotional outbursts, but Eugene was special.

Ping pong is a game of action and reaction. Conceptually, it was the perfect fit for Eugene's personality. Whether Eugene won a point or lost a point, he always had a predictable reaction. If he won a point, he would let out a high-pitched and gleeful, "C'mon!" His parents would clap, holler, and cheer him on. If Eugene lost a point, he would put his hands on his hips and let out a higher pitched, and painfully drawn out, "Commme Awwwwwnnnn!"

These antics were always followed by a tremendous reaction from the audience. The entire stadium would erupt into thunderous applause, cheers, and even laughter. Eugene's opponent didn't matter. He was such a polarizing figure that table tennis crowds simply relished rooting *against* him. Wherever he played, crowds followed.

It was no different that summer in 1988, when I found myself competing for the coveted gold medal at my first Junior Olympics. The whole tournament had been a whirlwind of an experience for me. So at the time of the final match, I was totally naïve to the Eugene Huffington phenomenon. For all I knew, this crowd sure seemed to like me! Remembering how good it felt to have the support of the crowd later inspired me to be a vociferous cheerleader for my patients who were trying to win at weight management.

Eugene won the toss and elected to start serving. He held out his extended arm, tossed the ball in the air, and the match began. I mishandled my service return and Eugene won the first point. His parents gave him a standing ovation, while the rest of the stadium stayed deathly silent. He served again and we got into a rally, like two boxers throwing punches, until another ball whizzed by me and, just like that, I was down two to zero. Eugene's parents were ecstatic. I could feel the expectant eyes of the rest of the crowd bearing down on me.

In despair, I looked at my family for some support. I saw my dad, who got me interested in the sport and acted as my first coach. Despite his busy professional life, my dad devoted countless hours teaching me the basics of ping pong, improving my mechanics, and shuttling me to and from tournaments.

I looked at my mother, the yin to my dad's yang. Her easygoing nature has always balanced my dad's stubbornness. Their symbiotic relationship inspired the harmonious elements of the Ping Pong Diet.

I saw my brother, an important practice partner and a source of motivation and healthy competition.

Next to my brother stood Coach Hsu. Coach was built like an oak tree, with thick, defined branches for arms. Behind his wide-framed glasses was a stare that commanded complete authority. Coach Hsu took the sport of table tennis very, very seriously. When he taught me how to hit a forehand, he firmly grasped my hand and forced it through a football shaped motion. When he explained table tennis concepts, he pushed his words out with precision and bite, like a commanding officer sending his troops into battle.

Yet behind his intensity and passion for the sport lay softness and compassion for kids. Coach had a special talent not only for relating to kids, but also motivating them to do their very best. I owe him for pushing me to try out for the Junior Olympics, and giving me the confidence that I could succeed. I stole a glance at Coach and he reflexively exclaimed, "Gah yo!" This Taiwanese phrase translates literally to "add oil to the tank," and is a common phrase used when trying to encourage someone to muster up energy for pushing through a task.

Buoyed by the support of my team, I indeed found the fortitude to add oil to my tank. On the next service return, I took an exaggerated backswing and smashed a terrific forehand winner that whizzed right past Eugene. The whole stadium (minus Eugene's parents) erupted in a giant roar of approval. Eugene served another, this time toward my backhand side, and I pounced on the ping pong ball like a mouse on cheese. Again, I hit a clean winner and the crowd went nuts.

Back and forth it went, alternating between cheers from Eugene's parents and the chorus of cheers from the crowd at large. We traded serves every five points until the game was tied at fifteen all. A timeout was called, and we each ran to our contingent for moral and tactical support.

"Chris, you're doing great, but he is using your power against you!" explained Coach.

"His strength is his ability to block back whatever you give him at either wing. Don't play into his strength! Take his strength away from him! Jam him down the middle and force him to generate his own pace. Then, when he least expects it, you can hit a winner to the corner!"

Brilliant! As a player, sometimes it is hard to clearly break down your opponent's weaknesses. Often, all you need is an observant third party to point out an effective strategy to maximize your potential.

I went back to work, energized by Coach's advice. Unfortunately, it was Eugene's serve and he came back from the time out with his own agenda. He placed a carefully thought out slice serve to my forehand, applying backspin on the ball using a chopping motion. When I pushed the ball back, he continued to apply backspin directed at my forehand side. Clearly, his parents had figured out that I had difficulty with heavy backspins. Eugene was daring me to go on the offensive. I knew what his strategy was, but I refused to accept my own deficiencies.

I bent my knees, dropped my arm, and created a magnificent arcing motion—then promptly dumped the ball into the net. The next two points played out much the same. Suddenly I was down eighteen to fifteen, and three points away from losing the match. Three points ago, we were dead even. Now it seemed like I was at the bottom of a steep mountain. That's the psychological torture that comes from focusing on numbers and forgetting the big picture. I had worked too hard to just throw in the towel at this point! I stiffened my resolve, took a deep breath, and refocused myself.

I was determined not to make the same mistakes I had made in the previous points. Instead, I decided to exploit my opponent's weaknesses. Eugene served again but then I began dictating the point, countering with long, deep backspin shots of my own to the corners of the table. Eventually, Eugene tried to go on the offensive but misfired badly. Eighteen-sixteen. I applied the same strategy, and after a long rally, I got the same result. Eighteen-seventeen.

Now it was my turn to serve and I could dictate points from the start. I went right to work applying the strategy Coach had taught me. I sent a fast straight serve right down the middle, jamming up my opponent. He was able to block it back, but without much pace. I continued to jam him up the middle a few times, then crushed a forehand cross-court for a winner. We were all even now, and the crowd went crazy!

I applied the same tactics, then hit a sharp backhand down the line. Eugene lunged for the ball, but it ricocheted off the edge of his racquet and onto the floor. Just like that, I was up nineteen to eighteen. I could taste victory. Again, I served a missile straight up the middle, but Eugene was catching on to my strategy. He managed to put a bit more pace on his return, and we got into a rally. After several shots back and forth, my ball grazed the net and gently dropped onto his side of the table with an unceremonious ping. It never hurts to have a little luck on your side to get to match point. Somewhat embarrassed, I put up my hand in apology, but this only seemed to anger him more. On my next serve down the middle, Eugene shifted to the left, opening up his forehand to hit an out and out winner, making it twenty to nineteen.

A hush fell over the rest of the crowd. Suddenly I was back in my basement, doing drills alone with the green ball machine monster. All I could hear was the whirring of the machine and the rhythmic sound of ping pong balls being spit out like raindrops hitting a pool of water. I calmed myself. I thought about the moment and remembered myself. I realized I wouldn't win this match just by exploiting his weaknesses. Eugene had figured out my strategy and adjusted appropriately. In order to bring home victory, I had to rely on the complete game I had spent so many hours training to perfect. Instead of hoping my opponent would slip up, I needed to take control of this match and win it outright through my own efforts.

I served a side-spinning serve cross-court and we got into a gritty counter punching battle. I rolled a backhand cross-court and he blocked it back cross-court. I flipped a backhand down the line, and he looped a forehand wide cross-court. I dove after the wayward ball and managed a counter loop. He shot a forehand down my backhand side and I played a sweeping defensive slice that caught Eugene off guard. He tentatively pushed it back to me, and I took the opportunity to go on the offense, crushing a smashing winner. The crowd cheered in jubilation! I won!

I can remember being overwhelmed by both relief and a sense of accomplishment. I had set a goal, and thanks to my parents, my coach, the crowd, and myself, I got the job done. I won a gold medal at the Junior Olympics!

Chapter 2: Winning at Weight Management

Dieting can sometimes feel like a frustrating ping pong game. Many people who diet either simply can't lose the weight, or they watch helplessly as their weight goes back and forth again and again like a ping pong ball.

But ping pong doesn't *have* to be frustrating. Indeed, many kids are drawn to ping pong because it is a simple game anyone can play. One afternoon, I was at my parent's house with my two-year-old son, Colin. It had been more than a decade since I had last picked up a ping pong paddle, and I said to my dad, "How about a game?"

A faint smile came over my dad's face, "Sure!"

So we pulled out the old ping pong table, dusted off our paddles, and started hitting the ball around. Then I decided to get Colin into the act. I sat him on top of the table, placed a paddle in his hand, and guided him through the motions as my dad fed him balls, just like he did for me when I was a kid. "Ping," went the sound of the ball as it came into contact with his paddle. Colin squealed with delight.

It dawned on me that a primary reason most diets don't work is because they are too complex. No one wants to spend their days counting carbs and calories. So the Ping Pong Diet was designed to be so simple, anyone could pick it up and just do it—like a simple game of ping pong. Not only will I teach you a simple and effective strategy for weight loss, I will empower you with specific rules you can follow to keep the weight off. These rules are based on the proven success of people just like you who have been able to lose significant weight and maintain that weight loss. I have compiled these tips into an easy-to-follow twenty-one point plan for weight management.

And while they will give you the tools for great change, something has to drive that change. I can give you the keys, but you have to drive the car. Successful weight management is about successful *behavior* management. It is about discovering what drives your eating behavior, then controlling it. Ping pong taught me lessons applicable to life in general. I learned the value of hard work and commitment. I learned the importance of motivation and reward. But the greatest lesson I learned was that every one of us has the potential to win. The key is learning how to unlock that potential. And that is what this book is all about.

Weight management is one of the most gratifying things I do as an internist. Whether I'm helping a mother lose eighty-seven pounds for her son's Bar Mitzvah, or a father lose 147 pounds in anticipation of his son's birth, I have personally seen the power of harnessing human potential for incredibly meaningful change.

By far, my most successful patients have one critical thing in common. They are able to tap into their potential to win at weight management. The mindset of a successful weight manager is very much like that of an elite athlete. Both individuals need to set a personally meaningful goal and devote themselves to rigorous training of mind and body. Both individuals need to remain motivated and dedicated to achieving their long-term goals. As far off as that personal long-term goal may seem to you, consider this: Olympic athletes set a goal that is four years away. Just as athletes have coaches to support them through training, I will coach you through your weight management. The new habits I will introduce you to may feel foreign at first. But once these new habits become your own, you will become as masterful at managing food as a world-class athlete is at their sport.

In the end, who wins the gold medal? Is it the most talented athlete? Is it the athlete who spent the most money on expensive equipment and coaching? No. It is the athlete who wants it the most. In other words, if you want to be successful at weight management, you've got to be hungry for it! One of the most powerful tools for driving behavior is tapping into your competitive spirit to be your best. Just as an Olympic sprinter strives for faster and faster times, you can compete for your personal best. By tapping into your competitive drive, you can access your human potential to win. So I encourage you to think of yourself as an Olympic athlete. I encourage you to reach deep inside yourself and unlock your potential. I encourage you to find *your* gold medal moment!

Chapter 3: Nobody's Body but Yours

Michael Phelps was having a spectacular 2008 Summer Olympics. But midway through the 100 meter butterfly, his prospects for achieving a record-setting eight gold medals in a single Olympics looked dismal. After fifty meters, he was seventh in an eight-man field. Then he turned it on. As the crowd cheered, Phelps closed the gap until there was only one man to beat—Milorad Cavic. With less than a meter to go, Phelps still visibly trailed Cavic as Cavic glided toward the wall for what seemed like an inevitable win. However, in the final moments, Phelps mustered another half stroke, stretched his arms, and touched the wall 0.1 seconds before Cavic. In doing so, he accomplished a seemingly impossible physical feat, and tied Mark Spitz's record of seven gold medals in a single Olympics.

An athlete is defined as a participant in a sport or game requiring physical skills such as agility, stamina, or strength. Elite athletes like Michael Phelps develop such masterful control of their bodies, they almost seem able to defy space and time. To become like an elite athlete, you will also need to develop masterful control over your own body. Like an elite athlete, you'll need to know how to take care of your body so you can perform at your highest level.

Excess weight literally weighs you down. It wreaks havoc on your health. For instance, excess weight, particularly belly fat, is associated with a greater risk of high blood pressure, elevated blood cholesterol, diabetes, and even fatal heart disease. Research indicates belly fat is not an inert energy depot. It is actually an active organ emitting hormonal signals that negatively impact health. Like an invisible radio wave colliding and interfering with the transmission of your Wi-Fi signal, belly fat secretes hormones that disrupt normal metabolism and result in damaging inflammation.

All that damage takes a toll on your body, preventing you from feeling and performing optimally. It is like a car needing an oil change badly—except the build-up I'm talking about may ultimately lead to a heart attack! Weight loss dramatically improves health by reversing derangements in blood cholesterol and blood sugar. Weight loss is also associated with tremendous improvements in psychological well-being. People who lose weight often remark on how energetic and great they feel. That is how being a lean, mean, well-oiled machine feels!

To become like an elite athlete, you'll want to first get rid of any excess weighing you down. But exactly how do you do that? You might assume the key to a lean, healthy body is spending hours at the gym. Well, it isn't. In fact, studies show that exercise results in an average weight loss of only three-and-a-half pounds.[1]

Exercise is **NOT** an effective strategy for weight loss! To learn how to sculpt your body into a lean machine, you must first understand how your body evolved to survive. Our bodies are the result of millions of years of evolution. Energy, in the form of food, means survival for a species. But over the course of human history, food has not been as plentiful as it is today. Humans had to survive through famine, war, and scarcity of resources. Over time, human bodies became highly efficient at utilization, conservation and storage of energy. If exercise were so effective at burning calories, our prehistoric ancestors would have withered away to nothing running away from wooly mammoths and saber toothed tigers! On the contrary, your body is built to conserve as much energy as possible during exertion, and store as much energy as possible at mealtimes.

Your body isn't designed to face the likes of our twenty-first century diet! The modern diet is so full of foods that efficiently turn into body fat, that two-thirds of Americans are now either overweight or obese. So how can you effectively lose weight in the twenty-first century? The first step is eliminating what caused the problem in the first place—nutritionally poor and fattening processed foods.

The second step is realizing your body can get the energy it needs from either the outside, when you consume food, or from the inside. The food you bring into your body from the outside is not just a tasty treat. First, food is an important source of essential micronutrients and macronutrients, including vitamins, minerals, essential fats, and amino acids. Your body cannot manufacture essential nutrients. They must come from your diet, and are necessary for normal function and metabolism.

Second, food is a source of energy through the three macronutrients—carbohydrates, fats, and protein. Your body uses carbohydrates (grains, fruit, beans, dairy, and vegetables), fats (in meat, butter, nuts, avocado, etc.), and protein from animal or plant sources for energy.

Third, food communicates certain messages to your body. Eating regular amounts of carbohydrates tells your body that outside food is plentiful, diverting it from tapping into its own fat stores for energy. Alternatively, restricting carbohydrates says outside food is scarce, directing your body to burn its fat stores for energy.

Let me explain a little further. Although your body can use protein as an energy source, under normal conditions, it mainly burns two types of fuel for energy—carbohydrates and fats. It typically alternates between burning primarily carbohydrates for fuel during meals (assuming the meals being eaten contain some carbohydrates) and burning primarily fats for fuel between meals and during sleep.

Furthermore, the amount of carbohydrates going into your body dictates whether you burn fat or carbohydrates for fuel. As you increase carbohydrates in your diet, carbohydrate burning goes up and fat burning goes down. And as you decrease carbohydrates in your diet, carbohydrate burning goes down and fat burning goes up. One way to think of this is that your body is set to burn fats unless rudely interrupted by a meal with carbohydrates.

Therefore, the key to maximizing weight loss is to lower your carbohydrate intake so that your body will be forced to burn fat for energy…your fat! The efficacy of carbohydrate restriction for weight loss has been demonstrated in multiple studies.[2, 3] You may even know someone who lost significant weight using a low carbohydrate diet. In fact, compared to other dietary strategies, carbohydrate restriction results in less hunger, greater satisfaction, and twice as much weight loss![4]

Now that you understand the basis for how your body works, what do you want for your body? Do you want your body languishing in a pool of diabetes and heart disease? Or do you want to learn how to master your body like an elite athlete? Now, who's ready for some ping pong?

Chapter 4: The Ping Pong Diet

Vegetarians and vegans say, "Eat plants." People in the Atkins and Paleo camps say, "Eat meat." Who's right? Both! The health promoting power of plants and protein are not mutually exclusive. In fact, plants and protein have a symbiotic relationship for weight management and health. Just as ping pong is a game of symmetric halves, the Ping Pong Diet, or PP Diet, provides you with nutritional symmetry. The first "P" of the PP Diet stands for plants—specifically, nonstarchy vegetables. The second "P" stands for protein—specifically, lean protein.

Plants are the yin to protein's yang. For instance, an exclusively vegetarian diet lacks vitamin B12. On the other hand, an exclusively meat-based diet lacks vitamin C. Together, plants and protein give your body all the essential vitamins and minerals it requires for normal functioning and metabolism. Also, an exclusively vegetable-based diet lacks essential fats and amino acids. The lean protein in the PP Diet provides a complete source of essential amino acids, as well as small amounts of the essential fats required to thrive. Finally, plants and protein chemically balance each other out. Higher protein intake tends to shift blood chemistry toward a more acidic state, while higher plant intake tends to shift blood chemistry toward a more alkaline state. Eating *both* protein and plants keeps your body neutral, and that is when it is happiest, at least chemically speaking.

Not only do plants and protein give you all the nourishment your body needs, this combination of nutrients is key for effective weight loss, and weight maintenance. Plants and protein fill you up without filling you out. That is why the PP Diet is made up of exclusively plants and protein. The PP Diet is as easy as eating two cups of vegetables and a serving of protein the size of a deck of cards, five times per day. It's really that easy! Surely you can do that. Now, let's look at the plan in detail.

Plants: Eat Two Cooked Cups, Five Times Per Day

While you are on the PP Diet, you will be eating vegetables—a lot of vegetables! Think fresh, flavorful, and filling! Any nonstarchy vegetable, such as zucchini, spinach, peppers, mushrooms, lettuce, arugula, asparagus, cucumber, cabbage, bell peppers, broccoli, celery, cauliflower, eggplant, tomatoes, collards, mustard greens, watercress, bok choy, swiss chard, escarole, and kale, just to name a few, is recommended. Dark green, leafy vegetables like spinach and kale are particularly good sources of essential vitamins and minerals.

Because nonstarchy vegetables are very low in carbohydrate density, you can fill up on a large quantity of them and still lose considerable weight. But you will also need to purposefully restrict all other carbohydrate sources, including:

- Sugars, sugary beverages, and processed foods

- Alcohol

- Starches (bread, pasta, rice, cereal, flour)

- Starchy vegetables (onions, brussels sprouts, artichokes, okra, potatoes, sweet potatoes, yams, taro, beets, turnips, parsnip, carrots, plantains, winter squash, pumpkin, peas, corn, and corn starch)

- Fruits

- Beans

- Dairy (milk, cheese, yogurt, ice cream)

- Nuts

There is no need to count carbohydrates while on the Ping Pong Diet. Just eat two cups of cooked (or four cups raw) nonstarchy vegetables, five times per day. Eating five times a day is an essential strategy to curb hunger and reduce the chance of eating outside the plan.

One of the most critical points to learn about effective weight *loss* (weight maintenance is an entirely different animal) is that carbohydrates are carbohydrates. Even good carbohydrates like fruit, beans, nuts, whole grains, and low fat dairy, which are great for weight maintenance, have too many carbohydrates for the purpose of weight loss, and are therefore restricted while you are on the PP Diet. However, keep in mind that they will be reintroduced during your transition phase, and continued during maintenance.

Protein: Eat One Deck of Cards Five Times Per Day

The Ping Pong Diet is also high in protein, matching protein intake with carbohydrate intake in an approximate 1:1 ratio. Studies show higher protein intake is associated with significantly higher weight and fat loss.[4, 5] For example, increasing the percentage of protein intake from 15 percent to 30 percent, while keeping carbohydrate intake constant at 50 percent, has been shown to result in reductions in hunger, spontaneous eating, body weight, and fat.[5]

Although you may have heard that high protein diets are unsafe, protein intake as high as double the recommended amount has been demonstrated to be safe in clinical studies. However, because high protein intake can predispose to kidney stones, you should aim to drink eight glasses of water per day on this plan. In other words, hydrate till your pee-pee is clear while you are on the PP Diet! High protein diets are not recommended for those with preexisting kidney failure.

Pair your vegetable intake with one serving of protein the size of a deck of playing cards five times per day. Eat protein from a variety of sources (seafood, chicken, pork, and beef) to ensure you get all essential vitamins, minerals, and amino acids. In addition, make sure to eat fish (preferably wild-caught) twice a week, and cook with up to two tablespoons of canola oil each day to get your essential omega-3 fats.

One notable way the Ping Pong Diet differs from other low carbohydrate diets is the protein eaten on this plan is low in fat. When choosing meat, ignore the misleading term "lean", which is displayed on the front of the package. Lean content is calculated by weight, which includes the weight of water. Instead, look at the nutrition label located on the back of a package of meat, and choose only meats with one-third or less fat content by *calories* per serving. For instance, if the nutrition label says 150 total calories and 100 calories from fat, you would not select that cut of meat. However, if the nutrition label says 150 total calories and fifty calories from fat, that would be considered a lean protein acceptable on this plan.

Vegetarians can also follow the PP Diet, but the visualization tool using a deck of cards to indicate protein serving size would not apply. Instead of a serving of meat the size of a deck of cards, vegetarians can eat six egg whites or three-fourths cup of EggBeaters five times a day. For the purposes of weight loss, egg whites are preferable to whole eggs because the white part of the egg is pure protein. Of special note, although eggs are found in the dairy aisle of your grocery store, eggs are protein, not dairy since they don't come from the mammary glands of mammals. Another option for vegetarians is to use veggie burgers (i.e., MorningStar Farms) as their source of protein. However, because veggie burgers contain carbohydrates, the amount of nonstarchy vegetables needs to be reduced. For every patty of MorningStar veggie burger eaten, the amount of cooked nonstarchy vegetables should be reduced by one cup. On this plan, a vegetarian that uses MorningStar veggie burgers as their source of protein would eat one MorningStar veggie burger patty and one cup of cooked nonstarchy vegetables five times per day.

More Than Just a Diet

The PP Diet is much more than just a diet. By embracing the power of plants and protein, the PP Diet teaches you to conceptualize food in an entirely different way. It teaches you that you can give your body all it needs while enjoying fresh, flavorful, and filling food. Enhance the flavor of your foods naturally with salt and chicken broth. Use black pepper, red pepper flakes, and other spices to add heat. Add acid like lemon and lime juice to bring out the brightness of your food. Add depth to your flavor profiles by using fresh herbs like parsley and basil. Eat fresh vegetables and try simple cooking methods like roasting to bring out the natural sweetness of your vegetables. By cooking fresh, flavorful, and filling food, you will awaken your taste buds, and gain a whole new appreciation for food. To get started, try some of the recipes listed at the end of this book.

Like an elite gymnast who has complete control on a balance beam, the PP Diet helps you take control over physiological hunger. Have you ever eaten a bagel, then three hours later, you are suddenly overcome with sweats, shakes, and hunger? That is your body's hormonal response to the bagel leaving your system. Most of us respond to that feeling by wolfing down something sweet, like a donut or cookie, thus creating a vicious cycle I call the carbohydrate rollercoaster.

When you start a low carbohydrate plan such as the PP Diet, you are drastically changing the way your body uses fuel sources. Instead of a cyclical pattern of eating sugars and carbohydrates, you change the way your body uses resources for energy. When you start the PP Diet, your body will first make use of short-term carbohydrate stores such as glycogen. As your blood sugar level declines, your body will send off alarm bells in the form of stress hormones like adrenalin and cortisol to help keep your blood sugar level in a normal range. These stress hormones are responsible for symptoms such as hunger, shakiness, cramps, dizziness, fatigue, headaches, and irritability—the same type of symptoms you get three hours after eating a bagel.

You will likely feel the urge to grab a sugary carbohydrate from the restricted list. Don't do it! Doing so will sabotage your plan, and prevent you from getting into fat burning. If you continue to follow the plan, you can expect these symptoms to dissipate after three to five days. After this initial phase, you will deplete your glycogen stores and get into consistent fat burning. Not only will your symptoms subside, but you may actually feel more energetic. Additionally, most people also experience a reduction in cyclical hunger after getting off the carbohydrate rollercoaster. Most of my patients who have tried the PP Diet say they don't feel hungry anymore. In fact, patients complain there is *too much* food on this dietary plan. Using the PP Diet will help you control your hunger so you are no longer powerless when it comes to food; instead you will find food to be empowering. Suit up and get in the game! Let's eat!

Chapter 5: Weight Loss Versus Weight Maintenance

Congratulations on making the decision to get in the game and try the PP Diet! You are probably losing weight already. And while the decision to compete is the most critical step toward becoming an elite athlete, it is only the first step in a lifelong commitment to yourself and your health. Too often, diet books focus on the reasons why you should lose weight, and culminate with their plan for weight loss without teaching you how to keep the weight off. Therefore, even if readers do manage to lose weight, most fall back into old habits and regain the weight.

This book is structured entirely differently. My philosophy is to *do* what works for weight loss while you *learn* what works for maintenance. That way, all your hard work to lose weight will not be for naught.

When I set the goal to win a gold medal in the Junior Olympics, I began a training regimen for the event one year beforehand. That training consisted of regular practice with my brother, drills with my coach, games with my dad, tournaments, and even ping pong camp. The ultimate goal was to be the best ping pong player I could be, not just to win a gold medal. After I returned home from the Junior Olympics, I didn't just stop my training. I continued putting in the time to improve and maintain the skills I had worked so hard to acquire. What many people don't realize is an athlete might work on certain drills to get to an elite level, and a totally different set of drills to maintain that elite level of play.

A lot of people come to me for weight management after multiple failed attempts at losing or maintaining weight loss. Many people try very hard to make healthy eating choices, but they don't understand why eating healthy doesn't lead to substantial weight loss. When I recommend the PP Diet for weight loss, they are often surprised that certain healthy foods like fruit, beans, and whole grains are initially excluded.

Even when people have had success at losing weight, they often struggle to keep the weight off. Some become so defeated, they resign themselves to believing they will always be overweight.

The single biggest problem with dietary advice for weight management is not clearly differentiating what is effective for weight loss versus what is effective for weight maintenance. There are some universally effective principles that apply to both weight loss and weight maintenance, but often, what is essential for one is not for the other, and vice versa. Some of the principles that apply to weight loss, weight maintenance, or both are illustrated in the following table:

Weight Loss	Weight Maintenance
Very low carb	Moderately low carb
Quantity of carbs	*Quality* of carbs
Vegetables essential	Vegetables essential
Higher protein	Higher protein
Fiber preferable	Fiber essential
Low fat preferable	Low fat essential
Grains excluded	*Whole* grains
Sleep essential	Sleep essential
Exercise *not* essential	Exercise essential

The distinction between principles of weight loss and principles of weight maintenance is absolutely *critical*. Don't get creative while you are in the weight loss phase. Just continue the principles of plants and protein for maximal weight loss. While you are following the PP Diet, I will teach you the twenty-one point plan for weight maintenance. That way, once you reach your goal weight, you will know exactly how to keep it off.

Some people criticize low carbohydrate diets because they believe fast weight loss inevitably leads to regaining all the lost weight. Indeed, our bodies are hardwired to maintain homeostasis. For instance, if I turn the temperature down in the room you are sitting in, you will automatically start shivering to increase kinetic energy and raise your body temperature. Likewise, if you go on a diet, your body recognizes an energy deficit, and responds with compensatory mechanisms that promote weight gain.

But this doesn't mean you should give up trying to lose weight. What it does mean is proactively learning the behaviors and tools effective for weight maintenance while you are losing weight is critical. By properly planning and learning about effective weight maintenance strategies while you are losing weight, you minimize weight regain and achieve long-lasting health. This way, you can go from dieting to dominating! Over the course of the rest of the book, I will guide you through a twenty-one point plan for weight maintenance that's as easy as a game of ping pong.

Chapter 6: E-stablish a Routine

Your twenty-one point plan to go from dieting to dominating can be remembered using a very simple mnemonic: EAT WELL, BE WELL, FEEL WELL! It stands for:

1. Establish a routine

2. Avoid the attack of processed foods

3. Television leads to tele-tummies

4. Water: an essential nutrient

5. Eight hours of sleep

6. Label literacy

7. Low fat intake

8. Breakfast: the meal of champions

9. Eat frequently

10. Weigh yourself

11. Encouragement: adding oil to your tank

12. Lower your glycemic index

13. Limit sugars and sugars in disguise

14. Fiber

15. Eat your veggies

16. Exercise

17. Lean protein means lean you

18. Whole or not at all

19. Eating system for transition and maintenance

20. Learn to master your mind

21. Live!

When I was training for the Junior Olympics, I spent one to two hours a day playing ping pong. The format of my training always followed the same pattern. I started off with some stretches, did ten minutes of warm up, cycled through drills involving all the basic strokes, then finished up with game simulation. In the rare instance my coach or dad wasn't available, I would hit with the green ball machine monster. This unforgiving contraption relentlessly spits out balls at various spins and speeds. Returned balls are subsequently snared in its return tray and sucked up. Then the cycle begins anew.

Although somewhat monotonous, the routine I established was essential to creating a habit that would eventually take me all the way to the podium at the Junior Olympics. In his book, *Outliers*[6], Malcolm Gladwell writes about the "ten-thousand-hour rule." The premise of the ten-thousand-hour rule is that regardless of talent, achieving mastery requires thousands of hours of practice.

Establishing a routine is a critical strategy for lifelong weight maintenance. A routine is simply practice time. As you put in more and more practice time, you gradually change your behavioral pattern until you perfect a new habit. The mind is a very powerful thing, and just as you can develop bad eating habits, you can retrain your mind to adopt new, healthy habits. In *The Power of Habit*[7], Charles Duhigg writes:

"And once you understand that habits can change, you have the freedom—and the responsibility—to remake them. Once you understand that habits can be rebuilt, the power of habit becomes easier to grasp, and the only option left is to get to work:"

A habit is simply an evolutionary mechanism for a learned task. As you form a new habit, you become quicker and quicker at performing that given task. This allows you to expend less mental energy on the task, and eventually, performance of the task becomes automatic.

Charles Duhigg continues:

"MIT researchers discovered a simple neurological loop at the core of every habit, a loop that consists of three parts: a cue, a routine, and a reward."

To change your habits, Duhigg describes four steps: identify the routine, experiment with rewards, isolate the cue, and finally, have a plan. In other words, to change your habits, you need to first start by analyzing your habit loop. You can then make a plan to replace those unhealthy habits with healthy ones and make them your new routine.

I applied this concept to help my toddler, Colin, adopt a new habit. Now, my son is absolutely adorable. He really is. But when he's trying to learn a new skill, like getting potty-trained, he's not so adorable. In fact, I vividly remember crouching on a dirty restroom floor in Chipotle trying to coax the shit out of him. Literally. Initially, it wasn't clear if my son had any clue what my wife and I were trying to teach him. All he knew was, "Shit happens." Then he would run off and play.

So my wife and I identified the routine: he habitually shat in his pants. Isolating the cue was easy enough, since his face turned beet red and he started grunting in the middle of the living room. However, teaching him to understand the cues his body gave him was a bit more challenging. Each time we sensed he was starting to push, we rushed him into the bathroom, sat him on the potty, and waited. Nothing. But we persisted. Then one day, he pushed out a single golden nugget. My wife and I immediately congratulated and rewarded him. From then on, we experimented with rewards varying from stickers to watching a video. My wife came up with an ingenious "reward box," where Colin could choose his reward after going to the potty. He began learning his body's cues and changing his habits, and eventually he no longer needed external rewards, but instead relied on the self-satisfaction of a job well done. Yes! My son achieved continence!

These methods are applicable to your weight management as well. In the weight management classes I teach, I have the great fortune of working alongside a gifted cognitive behavioral psychologist, Dr. Stewart Zelman. In *THINK*[8], Dr. Zelman describes a behavioral pattern he commonly observes among individuals with eating problems. He writes,

"Over-eaters, for example, frequently head straight for the kitchen after work...they come through the front door, grab their mail, walk into the kitchen, open the refrigerator, and snack. After their snack they will change clothes or wash up after work. It is difficult to change patterns because they have become embedded habits, neurologically built in. How can we change a behavior pattern or create a new habit? In this example, I would suggest that when that person walks into the house, she go immediately to the bedroom and change her clothes, or come in through a different door. That break-up of the pattern allows her to go on with the rest of the evening without

needing a snack, and without opening the snacking behavior pattern."

In this example, the behavioral pattern drives hunger and eating instead of vice versa.

Establishing your routine for weight maintenance begins with breaking old, damaging dietary habits and adopting new, positive ones. New habits don't happen overnight. It takes work and conscious effort initially. But once new habits become your new routine, they unconsciously become automatic. A food journal is a great way to force new habits into your consciousness by making you aware of your food intake.

Another great habit is to plan out all your meals and snacks ahead of time. A significantly greater number of successful weight maintainers use this strategy. Take the routine of planning you have already developed by following the Ping Pong Diet and make meal planning your new habit. By establishing a routine, you change the neural patterns in your brain, and before you know it, you become masterful at your own weight management!

Chapter 7: A-void the Attack of Processed Foods

Whether you realize it or not, you are under attack. And you have been for some time. Look left, and you are accosted by a processed food industry accounting for $1 *trillion* in sales per year in the United States. Look right, and you are bombarded by a food industry that spends egregious amounts of money on advertising, second only to the automobile industry. It's become so bad that food manufacturers now spend nearly twice as much money on advertising their cereals as they do on the ingredients that go into them. Look all around, and you are surrounded by a fast-food industry that is so omnipresent, American spending on fast food went from $6 billion to $110 billion annually in the last thirty years alone. Look above, and you are victim to an aerial attack of misguided dietary guidelines and government subsidies, like those for milk fat and high fructose corn syrup production that worsen your health.

In order to win at weight management, you need to learn about your opponent. You need to understand how your opponent attacks you, so you can properly defend yourself. When I was playing in the championship match, any time I let Eugene dictate the shots, I was no better than a puppet on strings. Instead of dominating, I was allowing myself to be dominated.

When it comes to weight management, your primary adversary is not food or food excess in a general way. Your opponent is processed food. Specifically, packaged food with added sugars or processed carbohydrates that act just like sugar. Examples include certain snack foods (i.e., cookies, cakes) and processed starches (i.e., breads, ready-to-eat cereals, potato chips). These processed foods are particularly fattening because they are high in glycemic index.

Dr. David Jenkins introduced the concept of the glycemic index in 1981 to compare the rise in blood sugar after eating various carbohydrates. As a standard reference point, he assigned a value of 100 to the degree of blood glucose elevation after eating a fifty-gram carbohydrate load of pure glucose. He then fed an equivalent load of carbohydrate from a variety of cooked foods to healthy volunteers after an overnight fast, and measured the subsequent rise in blood glucose. The glycemic index of a given food was calculated based on the percentage rise in blood glucose relative to the reference standard. For instance, if the elevation in blood glucose from eating fifty grams of black beans compared to fifty grams of pure glucose is 30 percent, then the glycemic index of black beans is determined to be thirty. In general, foods with a glycemic index greater than fifty are considered high in glycemic index.

One of the most important discoveries Dr. Jenkins made was that two foods made up of equivalent grams of carbohydrates may have vastly different physiological effects on blood sugar. Let's take a typical value meal at your favorite fast-food joint—the epitome of a processed meal. The buns of most hamburgers are baked with refined flour, which is high in glycemic index. Do you want fries and a Coke with that? Soda is essentially high glycemic liquid sugar, whether sweetened by natural cane sugar or high fructose corn syrup. And the glycemic index of a raw white potato steadily increases as it is peeled, then boiled, then mashed, and finally reaches a level nearly equal to pure glucose when processed as a french fry. All that processing causes the sugars and carbohydrates in that value meal to be rapidly absorbed into your bloodstream. It's called fast food for a reason!

Studies show that eating a high glycemic diet is associated with significant weight gain as well as unhealthy blood cholesterol patterns, a doubling in the risk of heart disease, and more than doubling of the risk for diabetes.[9-11]

Remember how carbohydrate restriction signals your body to go into a fat burning state? Well, eating a high glycemic index diet does just the opposite. Foods that spike your blood sugar turn on insulin, the hormone responsible for telling your body to go into a fat–storing state. Insulin diverts energy, in the form of sugar and fat, into your fat cells for storage. The higher your insulin levels, the more energy gets deposited into your fat cells, the fatter your fat cells get, and the more weight you gain. Individuals with insulin-secreting tumors called insulinomas secrete high levels of insulin independent of meals. These individuals invariably gain weight. Diabetics who take insulin shots to control their blood sugar also tend to gain weight. And regularly eating foods high in glycemic index is like giving yourself regular insulin shots!

The best defense against an attack from processed foods is to avoid those foods as much as possible. Some useful strategies include staying on the periphery of the grocery store where

unprocessed food is on display, shopping from a grocery list, or even employing home grocery delivery. Eat before social events, and bring healthy dishes to share at potlucks and dinner parties. When you do eat out, browse menu items in advance from home, choose restaurants that serve plants and lean protein, and avoid fast-food establishments. Compared to adults who reported eating at fast-food restaurants two or more times per week, adults who reported never eating at fast-food restaurants had higher odds of successful weight loss maintenance.

But while a stout defense against an attack from processed foods is essential, you can't just play defense. If you only play defense, the best result you can hope for is a tie. In my match against Eugene, I couldn't just block back his shots and hope he would let me win. If I wanted that medal, I had to go get it. And that is what I am teaching you to do in this book. You learn how to go on the offensive by developing new habits, and eating foods that will ultimately help you win at weight management!

Chapter 8: T-elevision Leads to Tele-Tummies

When I was a kid, my favorite television show was *The Wonder Years*. I could relate to Kevin Arnold's growing pains, awkward moments, fights with his older brother, and of course, experiences with unrequited love. I remember one Saturday morning, I was getting ready to sit down and watch my favorite show when my dad said, "Chris, I'm going grocery shopping. Come join me." I politely declined his invitation. My dad persisted, and I whined, "I want to watch my favorite television show! I don't want to go grocery shopping!" My dad was not happy with that response. In fact, he was livid. He stormed off by himself, while I was left to "enjoy" my program in silence. I sulked. How could I think about food when I was in the middle of watching television?

But that's the problem. People *can* and *do* think about food while watching television. In fact, multiple studies have demonstrated a positive association between hours spent watching television and overweight status. While this may not be a surprising finding, the reason for this might surprise you.

You might assume television watching is associated with weight gain because television watchers don't exercise. However, one of the great myths about body weight is that exercise, or the lack thereof, is the cure for, or cause of obesity. When it comes to body weight, food plays a far more significant role than exercise. In a study of over 50,000 nurses, watching more than forty hours of television per week was associated with a doubled risk of obesity and diabetes. And this finding held true across various exercise levels. Even physically active nurses gained weight if they watched a lot of television.

Interestingly, a number of studies have shown that food intake increases with television watching. For instance, one study found that college students ate more while watching thirty minutes of television when compared to listening to thirty minutes of classical music. Think about the last time you sat down to watch some television. Did you unconsciously start grazing on a snack? If so, was it because you were hungry or was it just force of habit? Mindless eating while watching television not only adds calories, it is a particularly fattening habit.

Another study found that adults who watched more than two hours of television per day snacked more and consumed more processed foods, like pizza and soft drinks, compared to adults who watched less than one hour of television per day. Not only do television watchers eat while watching television, they also tend to eat out more. The restaurant industry pays top dollar for all those commercials during your television program. They do so because it works. People who estimate watching three or more hours of commercials per day are more likely to report eating fast food for snacks or dinner than do people who estimate watching one or less hours of commercials per day.

But if watching television is associated with weight gain, can simply watching less television prevent weight gain? Yes! The National Weight Control Registry tracks over 10,000 individuals who have successfully lost at least thirty pounds and kept it off for at least one year. On average, registry members have lost sixty pounds, and kept the weight off for five-and-a-half years. One simple, but insightful, finding reported by this registry was that successful weight maintainers watch less television. While the average American watches twenty-eight hours of television per week, 62 percent of successful weight maintainers in the National Weight Control Registry watch less than ten hours of television per week. Instead of habitually sitting on the couch and watching television after dinner, establish a new routine! Read a book or go for a walk. Consider spending time with a loved one. Might I suggest a grocery trip with your old man?

Chapter 9: W-ater, an Essential Nutrient

What do you crave when you are thirsty? Psychologically, you may crave the buzz you get from drinking liquid sugar, but physiologically, your body just craves water. Your body is comprised of 60 percent water, making water an essential nutrient.

When I played ping pong competitively, I made sure to bring a bottle of water with me to keep up with fluid loss from sweating. Nowadays, advertisements prominently display elite athletes drenched in neon-colored sweat, chugging an equally neon-colored, sugary beverage to replenish their electrolyte and water losses. Indeed, cases of life-threatening dehydration, such as cholera-induced diarrhea, should be rehydrated with fluid containing sugar and electrolytes to maximize hydration. But most of us are not sweating to the point of life-threatening dehydration.

In the case of everyday life, sugary beverages are not only unnecessary, they are downright harmful. Sugary beverages such as sodas and fruit juices are a significant source of sugar in the American diet. In fact, one-third of added sugars in the American diet are hidden in the form of sugar-sweetened beverages. For example, a typical twelve ounce can of soda contains ten teaspoons of sugar in the form of high fructose corn syrup.

One of the problems with liquid sugar is that those calories are *added* to your meals. People do not compensate for sugar-sweetened beverages by reducing food intake. But sugary beverages are more than just added calories. Those additional liquid calories are particularly fattening because they are rapidly absorbed and have a high glycemic index. In the Nurse's Health Study, increasing consumption of sugary beverages from one drink per week to one drink per day correlated with a ten pound weight gain in four years and a near doubling in the risk of diabetes.

Those neon colored sports drinks are a particularly menacing problem. Sports drinks are typically high in both sugar and sodium. That sodium gets absorbed and simultaneously drags sugar into your body by acting on sodium-dependent glucose co-transporters lining your intestine. The net effect is rapid absorption of glucose into your body and subsequent fattening.

There's a famous saying, "There must be something in the water." That "something" is often sugar, and it's detrimental to your health. So, instead of drinking a sugar-sweetened beverage, make the choice to establish a new routine. Get in the habit of drinking water. It's calorie-free, and it's what your body really needs. For an added twist, try infusing your water with the natural essence of fruit and herbs. Whether at home, at a restaurant, or on the go, choose to make water your beverage of choice. Let's drink to your health!

Chapter 10: E-ight Hours of Sleep

"It's been a hard day's night
And I've been working like a dog
It's been a hard day's night
I should be sleeping like a log"

–The Beatles

The Beatles said it best. It *has* been a hard day's night. And you *have* been working like a dog. On top of that, you *should* be sleeping like a log. But when was the last time you actually had a good night's sleep? I mean a *really* good night's sleep? I credit a fantastic sleep medicine physician, Dr. Asefa Mekonnen, for educating me about the importance of sleep for proper health, and reminding me that sleep takes up approximately one-third of our lives. If you ignore the impact of sleep on your body weight and health, you are neglecting one-third of your life.

Just like food, sleep is a basic need of your body. When you don't eat well, your health suffers. Likewise, when you don't sleep well, your health suffers. Studies show that weight gain is related to sleep duration in a U-shaped distribution. Weight gain is higher for long and short sleep durations, and minimal with sleep durations in the middle of the distribution. What is that sweet sleep spot? Eight hours of sleep per night.

Why does an inadequate amount of sleep predispose to weight gain? Your body typically burns fats while you are sleeping. Sleep is an important time for your fat cells to get a little skinnier, and for your body to rectify some of the fattening that took place during the daytime.

Furthermore, people who spend less time sleeping and burning fat may simply be spending more awake time eating. In fact, sleep deprivation has been shown to drive overeating, particularly of fattening foods. For example, people who were given free access to meals and snacks ate significantly more snacks (i.e. pretzels, chips, crackers, muffins, cookies, candy, and ice cream) when they were sleep deprived. Another study found that compared to normal sleeping conditions, sleep deprived subjects reported a 33 percent increase in hunger for sweets like cakes, candies, cookies, ice cream, and pastries, and a 45 percent increase in hunger for salty foods like potato chips.

If adequate sleep is good for health and body weight, shouldn't longer periods of sleep be even better? Why are longer sleep durations associated with worse health outcomes and higher body weights? Longer sleep durations may be how your body compensates for poor sleep quality. Poor sleep quality can be a result of sleep fragmentation, where sleep is frequently interrupted throughout the night.

One prominent cause of highly fragmented sleep that is also highly associated with weight gain is sleep-disordered breathing. Do you snore? Snoring can be a symptom of sleep-disordered breathing involving disturbances to airflow and oxygenation. Obstructive sleep apnea (OSA) is the most common form of sleep-disordered breathing, and is strongly associated with weight gain. The prevalence of OSA among obese people has been reported to be as high as 50 percent! OSA is characterized by repeated episodes of decreased airflow accompanied by drops in oxygen levels or disruptive arousals from sleep. An individual with severe OSA stops breathing, or has a significant reduction in airflow, thirty or more times an hour. That's like being unconsciously nudged awake every two minutes, all night, by your spouse! It's not only annoying and disruptive, it's unhealthy.

So don't lose sleep over your weight. *Get* sleep to control your weight. Set a sleep schedule and stick to it. If you snore, or you feel excessively sleepy during the daytime, see a sleep doctor to get a sleep study checking for sleep apnea. That way, you can make sure to get eight hours of sleeping like a log. Sweet dreams.

Chapter 11: L-abel Literacy

Low! Reduced! Free! Less! These are just some of the many terms listed on processed foods that simultaneously inform, and confuse, most of us. Processed foods are products designed to sell, not to promote health. Clever packaging, misleading nutrition information, and manipulation of healthy buzzwords are techniques food manufacturers use to get you to buy their products and increase their profits. Rather than succumb to the creative ploys of food marketing, you can maintain weight loss and good health simply by significantly cutting down on (and, ideally, eliminating) processed food intake. Processed foods are often packed with added sugars or processed carbs that act just like sugar. They are also often high in sodium, which enhances the absorption of glucose into your body.

And, while avoiding processed foods and relying on whole foods like plants and protein are fundamentally important for successful weight maintenance, knowing how to read a nutrition label is an essential skill. By paying attention to nutrition labels, you take your game to another level, and outsmart the food industry.

Reading a nutrition label can sometimes feel like reading a foreign language. The trick is to block out all the useless fluff, and focus on what is important for weight maintenance. I don't use nutrition labels to tally calories or grams of carbohydrates over the course of a day. That's a headache. Realistically, who is going to keep track of these metrics every day for the rest of their life? I also don't use nutrition labels to calculate recommended intake of macronutrients based on a 2,000 kcal diet. That's arbitrary. A 2,000 kcal diet may or may not apply to you. And I certainly don't use nutrition labels to tabulate my intake of fiber, vitamin A, vitamin C, calcium, and iron. That's silly. Those nutrients should be incorporated naturally, through a diet of plants and protein, not from processed foods. Instead, I use nutrition labels to pick the healthiest brand out of a seemingly endless variety of options. In this chapter, I will cover the basics of label reading, and how to use labels to choose products lower in glycemic index. In the next chapter, I will discuss how to use labels to moderate your saturated fat intake.

Grab your favorite processed food out of the pantry and read along! Every nutrition label is organized in the same uniform manner. They all report total calories, total fat, saturated fat, sodium, total carbohydrates, sugars, fiber, protein, and a few vitamins and minerals. The most important thing to remember is that all of these quantities are based on the reported serving size, which is listed at the top of the label. It's also important to be aware that a serving may differ from what you actually serve yourself. For instance, you would think that a granola bar is one serving. However, one trick the food industry employs is to report a serving size as *half* of a bar. If you ate the whole bar, you would need to double all the nutritional quantities to obtain an accurate assessment of what you actually consumed.

By comparing total carbohydrates, sugars, and protein across brands, you can choose brands that are lower in glycemic index, and less fattening. Because protein lowers glycemic index, choose products lower in total carbohydrates and higher in protein. For example, if two granola bars of the same serving size have the same ingredients and total carbohydrates, then choose the one with higher protein content. A general tip is to pick foods with a 1:1 ratio or higher of protein to carbohydrates to offset the harmful effects carbohydrates have on weight.

For instance, a typical yogurt with fruit on the bottom contains twenty-eight total carbohydrates per serving, mostly sugars in the form of fermented milk sugar, fruit sugar, and high fructose corn syrup. It also contains six grams of protein in the form of whey. That's a pitiful ratio, with more than four times more carbohydrates than protein per serving. On the other hand, an identical serving of plain Greek yogurt contains only nine total grams of carbohydrates, but a whopping twenty-three grams of protein in the form of concentrated whey. That's a great ratio, with more than twice as much protein to carbohydrates per serving. That's why plain Greek yogurt is a fantastic choice for weight maintenance.

After total carbohydrates, nutrition labels are required to list how much of those carbohydrates come from sugars. Unfortunately, nutrition labels only have to list sugars in a general way, so often neglect to tell you how much *added* sugar, such as high fructose corn syrup, a product contains. These added sugars are the highest in glycemic index, and most harmful to your weight. There are plenty of examples of perfectly good, healthy carbohydrates food manufacturers have tainted with added sugar. These include sugared dried fruit, candied nuts, canned fruit in sugary syrup, or yogurt with fruit on the bottom. In order to distinguish between unsweetened products and products with added sugar, you need to compare the grams of sugar per serving across products.

For example, the nutrition label from plain yogurt may list seventeen grams of sugar in a one cup serving, while the label from vanilla-flavored yogurt may list thirty-four grams of sugar in a one cup serving. The sugar content in the plain yogurt is a combination of different types of fermented milk sugar, which are low in glycemic index, and healthy. On the other hand, the vanilla-flavored yogurt contains twice as much sugar—seventeen additional grams of unnecessary added sugar in the form of high fructose corn syrup or some other sweetener. In this case, "vanilla" is a euphemism for added sugar—four teaspoons' worth. By choosing the plain yogurt, you choose the lower glycemic option, and you choose to win at weight maintenance.

Congratulate yourself! You have taken a major step forward in your nutrition label literacy. See, reading can be fun.

Chapter 12: L-ow Fat Intake

You take the good, you cut the bad, and there you have the fats of life. Well, it's not exactly that simple. Indeed, dietary fat can be a confusing topic. Some of the confusion comes from the assumption that all fat is bad. Additional confusion comes from complicated and impractical dietary guidelines. Confounding the confusion are intentionally misleading food labels that disguise the true fat content of foods. In this chapter, I will give you a straight talk about the fats of life. I will then teach you about the role of low fat intake for the purposes of weight maintenance.

Up until now, I have emphasized that high glycemic carbohydrates drive weight gain by stimulating insulin and turning on your fat storage machine. Indeed, choosing low glycemic options is a critical strategy for successful weight maintenance. However, multiple studies have demonstrated that low fat intake is also important for successful weight maintenance. While high glycemic carbohydrates drive fattening, both carbohydrates and fats contribute building blocks for making your fat cells fatter. Additionally, your body preferentially burns up any available dietary sources of fat before it taps into your existing fat stores. In other words, you can't burn your existing fat stores if you keep on stoking the fire with cheesecake and hot dogs.

But not all fats are the same! A simple way of thinking about dietary fats is to break them out into the good, the bad, and the essential:

1. Eat your essential fats.

2. Cut out bad fats.

3. Substitute good fats for bad fats.

There are two sets of essential fats your body needs to function normally: linoleic acid and linolenic acid. Linoleic acid belongs to a family of fats called omega-6 fatty acids, while linolenic acid belongs to a family of fats known as omega-3 fatty acids. While both are essential, you should primarily focus on incorporating omega-3 fatty acids into your diet. The reason for this is that dietary sources of omega-6 fatty acids such as cooking oils are so abundant in the typical American diet, most people get enough of them even without trying. Also, boosting your omega-3 fatty acid intake is important, because a high ratio of omega-6 to omega-3 fatty acids in the diet is associated with inflammation and higher risk for many diseases, including heart disease and cancer.

On the other hand, a recent study showed that people with higher levels of omega-3 fatty acids in their bloodstream lived longer, and had less risk of fatal heart disease. Omega-3 fatty acids can be found in walnuts, flaxseeds, chia seeds, canola oil, and seafood. The richest source of omega-3 fatty acids is wild-caught fish. Because wild-caught fish eat algae, they are a better source of omega-3 fatty acids than farm-raised fish that are fed corn. Eating one to two six-ounce servings of fish per week reduces the risk of death by 17 percent, and risk of death from heart disease by 36 percent. Oily fish such as salmon, herring, sardines, and anchovies are particularly rich in omega-3 fatty acids. Also, these smaller fish are lower on the food chain, so they contain less mercury.

In order to understand steps two and three of my three-pronged approach, let's define what a good fat and a bad fat is. Good fats and bad fats differ in how many hydrogen atoms they contain. Fats with all their hydrogen atoms are called saturated, and are considered bad. With a few exceptions, saturated fats are found predominantly in animal products such as red meat, butter, milk, and cheese. Fats that are missing hydrogen atoms are called unsaturated, and are considered good. Monounsaturated fats have one hydrogen atom missing, and polyunsaturated fats have more than one hydrogen atom missing. Unsaturated fats are predominantly found in fish and plants such as olives, avocado, nuts, seeds, and plant-based cooking oils.

The point of going through the chemistry of fats is not to saturate your brain with worthless jargon, but to point out that fats are not all the same. For instance, unsaturated fats tend to be liquid, while saturated fats tend to be solid at room temperature. An unsaturated fat can become solid through a process called partial hydrogenation, which creates a trans fat. Foods made up of trans fats have an enhanced shelf life, because bacteria won't touch the stuff. Trans fats may be good for shelf life, but they're not good for you. Multiple studies have demonstrated that high trans fat intake is associated with higher blood cholesterol, and higher risk of heart disease. Trans fats are so bad, the FDA recently announced plans to completely ban them from our food supply.

The idea that saturated fat is bad and unsaturated fat is good is based on their opposite effects on bad blood cholesterol particles called Low Density Lipoprotein (LDL) particles. Research shows that LDL particles play a significant role in the development of artery-clogging heart disease. Saturated fats tend to raise LDL levels, while unsaturated fats tend to lower LDL levels. Studies show that reducing intake of saturated fat can reduce your risk of a heart attack by 14 percent. Additionally, *substituting* polyunsaturated fats for saturated fats is associated with as much as a 45 percent reduction in heart disease.

But do the terms good fat and bad fat extend beyond heart disease? Are bad fats more fattening than good fats and essential fats? Yes! For instance, animals fed good fats from canola or safflower oil gained less weight and body fat than animals fed bad fats from beef, even when total fat and caloric intake was the same. Additionally, one study found greater weight loss when subjects took fish oil supplements in addition to following a diet, compared to subjects who followed the same diet but took a placebo.

What explains the apparent different effects on weight between saturated and unsaturated fats? Unsaturated fats burn up faster than saturated fats. Furthermore, among the unsaturated fats, polyunsaturated omega-3 fatty acids are burned up fastest. Because unsaturated fats burn up faster, they are less prone to be stored as fat, and therefore less likely to contribute to weight gain than are saturated fats.

Based on this data, the second step of my three-pronged approach to fats is to cut out bad fats. Simple ways you can cut out saturated fats from your diet include avoiding processed foods, sticking to nonfat dairy, limiting red meat consumption to once per week or less, removing fat and skin from your meats, and avoiding fried foods.

One heavy source of saturated fats that often goes overlooked is ground meat. Most packaged ground meat has much higher amounts of fat than people realize. The confusion lies in the front of the packaging, which uses weight to describe the leanness of ground meat. Because meat contains water, and water has no calories, weight-based descriptions make the protein content seem much higher, and the fat content much lower, than they actually are.

For example, let's take a look at a package of ground beef advertised as 85 percent lean. Indeed, it is 85 percent lean and 15 percent fat by *weight*. However, that same package of ground meat actually contains more than 50 percent fat content when you calculate fat content by *calorie*. What about ground turkey? Turkey is considered a leaner source of protein, but you may be surprised to learn that even ground turkey can be fatty. For example, a package of lean ground turkey may be advertised as 93 percent lean and 7 percent fat content by *weight*. However, when you look at calories from fat, you realize that it, too, contains nearly 50 percent fat content by *calorie*.

Don't rely on misleading information on the front of meat packaging. Instead, read the nutrition label on the back, and follow my Rule of Thirds to reduce your saturated fat intake:

1. Divide fat calories by total calories, and choose meats with a ratio of one-third or less,

then,

2. Divide grams of saturated fat by grams of total fat, and choose meats with a ratio of one-third or less.

For instance, if your nutrition label says 150 total calories, and 100 calories from fat, you would put that meat right back on the shelf, because its ratio is two-thirds—much higher than what the Rule of Thirds allows. However, if your nutrition label says 150 total calories and fifty calories from fat, it would be considered a low fat item that passed the first criteria. But if that label says five grams of saturated fat and ten grams of total fat per serving, it would fail the Rule of Thirds due to a high saturated fat content. However, if that label says three grams of saturated fat and ten grams of total fat per serving, both criteria of the Rule of Thirds would be satisfied, and I would consider that product to be low in saturated fat.

Finally, the third step in my three-pronged approach to fats is to substitute good fats for bad fats. Instead of reaching for fatty processed snacks, grab a handful of nuts. Instead of cooking with butter, use up to two tablespoons of canola oil per day. Instead of steak, go fish. And instead of a bowl of ice cream, eat an avocado. OK, that last one is a bit of a tough sell, but you get the gist.

In the past two chapters, you learned how to read and you learned all about the fats of life. Now that you have acquired these basic life skills, let's take your training to the next level!

Chapter 13: B-reakfast: The Meal of Champions

The year was 1933. The World Series featured the New York Giants and the Washington Senators. The Senators put up a good fight, but in the end, the Giants' pitching proved too tough for the Senators, and the Giants won the series in five games. The Giants earned the right to call themselves champions.

The Giants weren't the only champions from that year. That was also the year General Mills came up with their now famous slogan, "Wheaties—The Breakfast of Champions." Since the inception of that winning slogan, countless athletes, from Olympians to professionals, have graced the iconic orange Wheaties box. Catchy, memorable, and inspiring, this bit of advertising brilliance grabs shoppers from the aisle and says, "I'm a champion. Eat like me and you, too, can be a champion!"

Likewise, if you want to win at weight maintenance, why not emulate those who are proven champions of weight management? Eighty percent of participants in the National Weight Control Registry reported eating breakfast daily.

You might assume that skipping meals is effective for weight control, because you're cutting down on your calories. But in the long run, it's a defective strategy. The problem is that skipping meals ultimately leads to bad decision-making the next time you do eat. Think about the last time you skipped a meal. You might not have noticed anything because you were caught up in your work. You may have even felt really productive because you saved time by skipping a meal, and got that much more work done. And then it happened. You got that gnawing feeling in your stomach. Soon, you felt dizzy. You began to feel almost as if your stomach was digesting itself. That is the feeling of hunger. Extreme hunger. What did you do? Did you calmly prepare yourself a healthy meal? Doubtful. When you skip meals, you pay for it later.

An interesting study entitled "First Foods Most," provides insight into the negative consequences of skipping breakfast. This study examined how fasting affected subsequent eating behavior. College students who fasted were three times more likely to start a lunch buffet with starches like bread rolls and french fries. Fasters were also two times less likely to start a lunch buffet with vegetables compared with college students who had eaten breakfast. All students—fasters and non-fasters, ate 50 percent more of the food item they started their buffet with. So, if you skip breakfast, you may be setting yourself up to ultimately eat more fattening carbs at your next meal.

Instead of skipping breakfast, commit to a simple habit of eating breakfast daily. This positive health habit starts your day off saying, "I'm in control of my food and my body!" Rather than leave your day to the whims of hunger, control your hunger within the first thirty minutes after waking by eating a proper breakfast.

What constitutes a proper breakfast? Most people would instinctively reply, "A healthy bowl of cereal." But that's the worst thing to have for breakfast! While breakfast is the meal of champion weight managers, ready-to-eat cereal is not actually the breakfast of champions. Many ready-to-eat cereals are high in glycemic index, due to added sugar or highly processed grains. Starting your day off with a bagel or a bowl of cereal washed down with a glass of orange juice is a surefire way of getting on a carbohydrate rollercoaster you won't ever be able to get off.

Instead of starting your day off with high glycemic carbohydrates, start each day renewing your commitment to PP—

plants and lean protein. Incorporating protein into every meal and snack you eat is a winning strategy for weight maintenance. That could mean eating a nontraditional meal featuring lean meat, like that from the Ping Pong Diet, for breakfast.

A great source of protein for breakfast is eggs. Eggs are rich in folic acid and vitamins A, E, and B12. Egg whites are an inexpensive, complete source of protein that can help with weight control. One study compared a weight loss diet of an egg breakfast versus a bagel breakfast in overweight subjects. After eight weeks, the egg group showed a 65 percent greater weight loss, and 34 percent greater reduction in belly fat, compared to the bagel group.

Another convenient protein-rich breakfast is nonfat plain Greek yogurt. Yogurt has been found to be inversely associated with weight gain. But not all yogurts are healthy! Avoid yogurts with added sugar, such as fruit-on-the-bottom yogurts. Plain Greek yogurt is especially good for weight maintenance, because it contains a high protein to carbohydrate ratio.

So emulate the behaviors of those with a proven track record of success. Start every day with breakfast—the meal of champions!

Chapter 14: E-at Frequently

The house was quiet—*too* quiet. And then I heard it...a rhythmic crunching sound. Out of the corner of my eye, I saw that the kitchen pantry door was ajar. I knew that *I* hadn't left it open. That could only mean one thing. I walked over and, of course, there was my son, Colin, gleefully munching away on a bag of potato chips. But how could I be upset with him? His body told him he was hungry, and he was resourceful enough to help himself to a snack.

Snacking is not only OK, it is an essential strategy for successful weight maintenance. The problem isn't that snacking is inherently an unhealthy behavior. The problem is that most conveniently available snack foods are processed foods that are unhealthy and fattening. The trick is not only embracing healthy snacking but scheduling eating occasions so you eat *before* you are hungry. That way, you won't let hunger control what you snack on.

While society dictates eating three meals a day as the norm, your body expects to be fed more frequently. For instance, my delightful toddler, Colin, lovingly demands to be fed approximately every three hours. This correlates with daily fluctuations in insulin levels and other appetite mediators that drive hunger. When you eat infrequently, you are more likely to allow hunger to overwhelm your decision-making. When you let your hunger control what you eat, you are much more likely to reach for fattening foods, and large amounts of them, as evidenced by the previously cited study, "First Foods Most."

Instead of letting hunger control what you eat, take control of your hunger by eating more frequently. One study showed that adolescent females who ate *more* frequently and snacked *more* frequently were *less* likely to gain weight or belly fat over a ten-year period. Indeed, compared to overweight individuals, successful weight loss maintainers and normal weight individuals eat more frequently, averaging about two snacks per day.

Incorporating two healthy snacks in addition to three regular meals per day translates into eating five times a day, or nearly every three hours. Eating more frequently not only controls hunger, it also helps keep blood sugar and insulin levels low, which minimizes fattening. For instance, one study showed that subjects who ate several smaller meals had 28 percent lower insulin levels compared to subjects who ate three large meals.

What constitutes a healthy snack for weight maintenance? Nonstarchy plants and lean protein are always excellent choices. However, vegetables and lean meat are not always convenient and handy. If I had to create the perfect snack, it would be a whole food that is portable, low in total carbohydrate and glycemic index, higher in fiber and protein, and not associated with weight gain. In a nutshell, I'm nuts about nuts! Studies have shown that nuts reduce hunger, and have an inverse relationship to weight gain. If used strategically, a handful at a time, nuts can serve as a great snack to help you control your hunger and win at weight maintenance.

So eat frequently and incorporate two healthy snacks a day. Not only will you control your hunger and maintain your weight, you won't be caught red-handed behind the pantry door munching away at potato chips.

Chapter 15: W-eigh Yourself

When I signed up for my first ping pong tournament, I went from being an unrated player to having an official USA Table Tennis rating. I was assigned a rating of 800, the equivalent of being a novice. After that, my rating increased whenever I beat a player with a higher rating, and decreased when I lost to a player with a lower rating. A player with a rating higher than 2,000 is considered to be an expert player.

This rating system served as an objective way of evaluating my progress as a player. It was also a source of significant motivation, bringing out my competitive spirit whenever I played someone with a higher rating. Having a rating also held me accountable, because I was always aware my rating would slip if I didn't remain consistent with my training.

Likewise, weighing yourself is a basic but important strategy for successful weight maintenance. Successful weight loss maintainers in the National Weight Control Registry reported that they frequently monitored their body weight. In fact, when successful weight loss maintainers are compared to counterparts who have regained weight, weight loss maintainers consistently report greater frequency of self-weighing.

All too often, and understandably so, people associate reaching their goal weight with crossing the finish line of success. Instead, I try to help people understand that all their hard work to reach a weight loss goal is for naught unless they make a lifelong commitment to health and weight maintenance as the ultimate goal. Commit to weighing yourself so you can catch small weight changes before large weight regain catches up with you. How often should you weigh yourself? I suggest checking in at least once weekly—75 percent of individuals in the National Weight Control Registry weighed themselves at least once a week.

And while objective self-monitoring is an important strategy for successful weight maintenance, it's important not to attach self-worth to a number on a scale. Weighing yourself too frequently, particularly in the weight loss phase, can be discouraging if the number reflected back does not meet your expectations.

When I started playing ping pong competitively, there was nowhere for my rating to go but up. Seeing that number steadily rise was thrilling! However, after a while, the incremental increases in my rating slowed. And in the later stages of my career, my rating plateaued in the mid-1,900s. How I longed to achieve a rating over 2,000 and be considered an expert player! I worked on my game, continued my training, and studied the games of top players, but despite my best efforts, I never got there. I realize now that, although it would have been nice to call myself an expert player, basing my self-worth on a rating scale was arbitrary. Incidentally, so is basing my self-worth on the number of visits to my blog (http://www.doctorchrisko.blogspot.com), YouTube channel (http://www.youtube.com/user/doctorchrisko), or website (http://www.mythicalweightloss.com), but now I'm getting off topic.

Likewise, your self-worth should by no means be measured by a number on a scale! The point of weighing yourself is not to torment yourself, but to empower yourself. Use the number to be proactive about small changes in your weight. It is much easier and healthier to actively manage your weight than to perpetually yo-yo from one extreme to another.

In addition to weighing yourself regularly, set an action weight. An action weight is a regain in weight that triggers action. I suggest 2.5 percent of your initial body weight. By setting an action weight, you avoid the slippery slope of "it's just one pound." In order to prevent one pound from becoming twenty, or even fifty, pounds, stop weight regain in its tracks! If you reach your action weight, examine your behaviors and make an honest assessment of what may have contributed to your weight regain. Go through the twenty-one points of weight maintenance, and identify where you may have taken a wrong turn. Reinvest yourself in the Ping Pong Diet, focusing on nonstarchy vegetables and lean protein to get back to your goal weight, and lock it in by recommitting yourself to your weight maintenance.

This type of proactive strategy is different from yo-yo dieting. A yo-yo swings wildly between extreme highs and lows. Yo-yo dieting implies lack of control. Instead, take control by weighing yourself and responding to small changes in your weight. Being attuned to your body, and precisely calibrating your body weight, is like being a master golfer putting his way to perfection.

So instead of dreading the weigh in, make sure you continually weigh in on yourself. Weighing yourself regularly can help you keep off the weight, and remain in tip-top form, so you can compete at your highest level.

Chapter 16: E-ncouragement: Adding Oil to Your Tank

Congratulations! You have reached the halfway point of your twenty-one point plan for weight maintenance. Now is a good time to pause and reflect on your progress. Have you taken pictures along the way? Have you been surprised by what you've been able to accomplish thus far? Take a moment to write down some things you are particularly proud of achieving. This is also a good opportunity to renew your commitment to yourself, and think about what motivated you to lose weight in the first place.

When I was training for the Junior Olympics, there were times that I just didn't want to play ping pong. There were times when I felt exhausted and frustrated. One of my favorite phrases was, "I can't do it!" This really irked my dad. He couldn't understand why my default mentality was so negative. I understood. Anything in life is easier if you simply conclude you can't do it. But then you don't get to actually show yourself what you are, indeed, capable of.

Perhaps you have had a day or two of frustration and disappointment. Perhaps the scale didn't tip your way, or you had a moment of indiscretion, went off plan, and are now beating yourself up about it. Although some people are able to focus on a task with robotic consistency, most of us have our human moments. But one day of frustration or indiscretion can easily lead to two or three days, and eventually you say, "I can't do it!" Rather than succumbing to negative mentality, it's critical to recognize that we all have those days. Instead of giving up, prop yourself up. Even winners need encouragement.

Encouragement can come from others, and it can come from within. Back when I was playing for a gold medal, I was blessed to have an incredibly supportive family and Coach. Although my coach wasn't a cuddly guy, he had a way of motivating me. Like dangling a carrot in front of a rabbit, Coach Hsu used to put candy on the edges of the ping pong table to motivate me and the other kids he taught. If you hit the piece of candy off the edge of the table, it was yours. Talk about brilliant. Incidentally, I do *not* recommend you try this at home for your own weight management. And whenever I was tired and dejected, Coach would tell me to "add oil" to my empty tank.

Just as competitive athletes fuel themselves with encouragement from others, you can excel at weight management if you surround yourself with support. Studies show that supportive group programs are more effective for weight management than individual counseling.

Some of the most powerful encouragement comes from those who care most about you. Engaging the support of your spouse or family member not only benefits you, it can change your entire home food environment for the better. For example, when patients of mine try the PP Diet, their spouses end up eating plants and protein by association. Can you guess what happens? They often lose weight, too! Another great source of encouragement is a friend who is also trying to lose weight. A friend who is struggling with their own weight can provide unique insight and supportive companionship. In fact, I *encourage* you to tell your friends about the Ping Pong Diet and play along together.

The most important kind of encouragement is the kind that comes from within. As supportive as a friend or family member can be, your weight management is ultimately your battle to win. Whenever you have one of those bad days where you tell yourself, "I can't do it," remind yourself of your goal, and the reason why you want to achieve that goal—your motivation. Your motivation can be positive, like wanting to look your best at your class reunion or wanting to climb Mount Everest. Alternatively, you may be motivated by the desire to avoid a negative outcome, such as diabetes or heart disease. But whatever the motivation, it has to be something deeply and personally meaningful to you. It has to make you *feel* something.

Visual imagery is a great technique you can use to stay motivated. Take pictures of yourself at periodic intervals. Comparing previous photos to current ones will help you create a visual map of where you once were, how far you have come, and how much closer you are to your final destination.

Don't forget to reward yourself along your journey. Setting short-term goals and incentives during your weight loss phase will help drive your behavior toward your long-term weight loss goal. Once you do reach your goal, don't forget to continue rewarding yourself for maintaining your weight. You could reward yourself with a new outfit or a massage every month you maintain your weight. How about a weekend trip, or a joy ride to a fun destination? You deserve it! You maintained your weight for three months. Just get the car and fill the tank to full. In doing so, you're not just adding oil to your car—you're adding oil to your motivational tank!

Chapter 17: L-ower Your Glycemic Index

The design of the Ping Pong Diet is to maximize weight loss and simplify eating by taking out all carbohydrates except nonstarchy vegetables. As you transition from a weight loss phase to a weight maintenance phase, you will want to reintroduce excluded carbohydrates, but be careful to select low glycemic options. Low glycemic eating minimizes your insulin secretion so fat storage and fat burning can be balanced.

Low glycemic eating consists of avoiding processed foods, and choosing low glycemic options among natural foods. In regards to processed foods, focus on eliminating packaged foods with added sugar or highly refined carbohydrates that act just like sugar. In regard to natural foods, be aware of starchy grains and root vegetables that tend to be high in glycemic index.

As a reminder, a glycemic index greater than fifty is considered high, while a glycemic index of thirty or less is considered low. Foods that are high in glycemic index are often high in carbohydrate count, but not always. Some foods that you avoided during your weight loss phase due to high carbohydrate counts are OK to eat for weight maintenance, because they are lower in glycemic index. These include onions, brussels sprouts, artichokes, and okra.

Nonstarchy vegetables and lean protein are low in carbohydrate count and glycemic index, so they are universally good for both weight loss and weight maintenance. For instance, zucchini, alfalfa sprouts, brussels sprouts, spinach, artichokes, bell peppers, peppers, arugula, broccoli, onions, asparagus, chives, mushrooms, fennel, leeks, lettuce, cucumber, celery, cabbage, and cauliflower all have a glycemic index less than fifteen, so are considered very low in glycemic index.

After nonstarchy vegetables, nuts and legumes are excellent choices during weight maintenance. For instance, most nuts and seeds, including pecans, almonds, walnuts, pumpkin seeds, and sunflower seeds, have a glycemic index around fifteen. Most legumes, including peanuts, soybeans, edamame, chickpeas, lentils, and black beans, have a glycemic index of thirty or less.

Most dairy products, like milk, are low to moderate in glycemic index. Fruits vary widely in their glycemic index. Most citrus fruits (i.e., lemons, limes, and grapefruit), stone fruits (i.e., apples, nectarines, peaches, and pears), and berries (i.e., raspberries, blackberries, and strawberries) are low in glycemic index. On the other hand, most melons (i.e., cantaloupe and watermelon) and fruits where the fiber is discarded (i.e., bananas and mangoes) are high in glycemic index.

As a category, starchy root vegetables and grains are higher in glycemic index. For instance, cooked starchy root vegetables like potatoes, sweet potatoes, yams, taro, winter squash, pumpkin, plantains, red beets, turnips, carrots, parsnip, peas, and corn, have a glycemic index greater than fifty. Pay special attention to avoid white potatoes, which are particularly high in glycemic index. For example, in a study looking at the weight gain potential of over fifteen categories of food, potatoes and potato chips topped the list at numbers one and two.

Grains such as bread, rice, and cereal are a prevalent source of dense carbohydrates that, in their natural state, have a moderate to high glycemic index. Processing of grains can further increase their glycemic index. Because processed grains are a major source of high glycemic carbohydrates, I will devote a dedicated discussion to this food group in the next chapter.

Choosing foods that are low in glycemic index is a critical strategy for successful weight maintenance. In one of the largest, most well-conducted studies on weight maintenance, people who lost at least 8 percent of their initial body weight were then randomized to weight maintenance diets varying by protein content and glycemic index. Over a twenty-six week period of maintenance, only the low protein/high glycemic index group regained significant weight. And, to no one's surprise, low glycemic eating was better than high glycemic eating at maintaining weight.

Various websites such as http://www.glycemicindex.com report the glycemic index of foods. While these serve as good guidelines, many factors can affect a food's glycemic index, including temperature, cooking duration, acidity, and of course, processing. Taken together, these factors can make your food act almost like pure sugar. Let's explore this further in the next chapter.

Chapter 18: L-imit Sugars and Sugars in Disguise

Back when we were cavemen and cavewomen, we used to consume twenty-two teaspoons of sugar per year. Now, Americans consume an average of twenty-two teaspoons of sugar per *day*. As discussed previously, one-third of added sugars in our diet come from sugary beverages. What about the other two-thirds? They're hidden…in your food.

Some common sweeteners include agave, molasses, honey, maple syrup, corn syrup, high fructose corn syrup, brown rice syrup, dark brown sugar, light brown sugar, date sugar, raw cane sugar, and sugar sugar. "You are my candy girl, and you've got me wanting you!" I've gone off topic. Regardless, all sweeteners are effectively sugar, because they all have the same physiological effects on your body. They are rapidly absorbed, cause abnormal spikes in your blood sugar level, and induce fattening through stimulation of insulin. Therefore, one of the most important things you can do to maintain your weight is limit your sugar intake.

Even less obvious than sugar pseudonyms, but no less harmful, are foods that don't taste like sugar, but act just like sugar in your body. These are carbohydrates that are so rapidly absorbed, and so high in glycemic index, that your body treats them like sugar. Many people already recognize that sweet rolls, cakes, muffins, and desserts are fattening. However, two of the most overlooked examples of sugars in disguise are processed bread and rice.

Bread, unhealthy? Blasphemy, you say! How dare I besmirch the name of the pillars of wheat that our great nation rests upon. Bread conjures up images of healthy, wholesome grains, so it's natural to assume that the processed bread loaves you buy at the grocery store are healthy for you. I'm here to tell you they aren't. Processed bread is not only one of the most overlooked examples of food processing, it is one of the most unhealthy things you can eat. On average, processed bread has a glycemic index of seventy-five!

In his book, *Wheat Belly: Lose the Wheat, Lose the Weight, and Find Your Path Back to Health*[12], Dr. William Davis argues that wheat is the single biggest contributor to the American obesity and diabetes epidemics. One of the most intriguing positions he takes is that all wheat products—even whole wheat bread—can be harmful.

The problem is particle size. Bread is traditionally made from coarsely ground flour. Now, modern commercial mills grind grains into very fine flour. This results in smaller particle sizes and an increase in exposed surface area during digestion. As a result, processed bread made from refined commercial flour is rapidly absorbed, regardless of whether it's made from white, brown, or 100 percent whole wheat flour. For instance, the average glycemic index of white bread is seventy-five and the average glycemic index of whole wheat bread is seventy-four. So don't be fooled into thinking you are choosing a healthy bread just because it is brown, or made from whole grains. Bread is the most prevalent example of high glycemic foods made from processed flours. Many other baked goods, like bagels, ready-to-eat cereals, pancakes, waffles, and pizza, are also made from refined commercial flour, and thus high in glycemic index as well.

That's why limiting your bread intake is a winning strategy for weight maintenance. If you do eat bread, I suggest limited quantities of sourdough or sprouted grain bread. Sourdough bread has a significantly lower glycemic index compared to other breads, around forty-eight. Sourdough bread is unique, because the sourdough starter has undergone a process of lactic acidosis by bacteria, which delays the absorption of the starch, and results in a lower glycemic index.

Even better than sourdough bread is flourless bread made from sprouted grains. Sprouted grain bread uses whole grains, such as wheat berries, that are soaked and allowed to germinate. These sprouted grains are then ground up, but not into fine flour. Because the whole grains are not ground into fine flour, bread made from sprouted grains is lower in glycemic index compared to other processed breads. Food For Life makes a line of sprouted grain breads that you can find in the frozen section of your local grocery store.

Another sticky and surreptitious sugar in disguise is rice. Just like bread, you can't judge a rice grain by its color. The average glycemic index of both boiled white rice and boiled brown rice is considered high, at seventy-three and sixty-eight, respectively. This might explain why one study found that substituting brown rice for white rice for sixteen weeks did not substantially affect blood sugar, weight, or waistline measurements.

Rice is comprised of starch granules that contain tightly packed chains of sugar molecules called amylopectin and amylose. Regardless of whether a grain of rice is white or brown, it undergoes a process called gelatinization when it is boiled in hot water. During gelatinization, the starch granules swell and the structural matrix is disintegrated, exposing the starch to digestive enzymes. This results in rapid digestion and absorption of the starch, with subsequent elevations in blood sugar levels.

Starch structure is more important than rice color. While all types of rice undergo gelatinization when boiled, rice grains that are comprised of higher amounts of amylose and lower amounts of amylopectin are digested more slowly, and have lower glycemic indices. This is because the compact linear structure of amylose molecules is less accessible to digestive enzymes than the branched structure of amylopectin molecules.

Short grain rice tends to be low in amylose, which results in stickier grains that are higher in glycemic index. On the other hand, the starch in long grain rice like basmati rice (common to Indian cuisine) is made up of a higher percentage of amylose. That's why cooked basmati rice grains tend to stay more separate, and have a lower glycemic index (forty-three) than other rice grains.

So take charge of your weight and your health by limiting sugars and sugars in disguise. Don't let food manufacturers determine how much sugar is added to your food. You should determine your own level of sweetness. Instead of obliging yourself to two slices of sugary carbs for lunch every day, skip the bread, and turn the inside of your sandwich into a generous salad topped with lean protein. Instead of a bed of rice, choose colorful vegetables as your base, and top with beans or whole grains. Now those are some *sweet* meals without the limitations!

Chapter 19: F-iber

"Beans. Beans. Beans. They're good for your heart."

That's a line from a catchy tune I loved to sing when I was a kid. OK, I still love to sing it to this day, even though I'm a grown man. But is it true? Are beans in fact good for your heart? Yes! In a study of Costa Ricans, eating one serving of beans per day was associated with reduced odds of having a heart attack. Large population studies also show that beans are associated with a 22 percent reduction in heart disease, and a 30 percent reduction in fatal heart disease.

Beans have an incredible nutritional profile; they are rich in essential vitamins and minerals, high in protein, and low in saturated fat and glycemic index. Part of the reason that beans have a low glycemic index is because they have higher amounts of amylose, the type of starch that is resistant to digestion. Beans contain 30–40 percent amylose, and 50–70 percent amylopectin in their starch granules, while most other starchy foods contain 25–30 percent amylose and 70–75 percent amylopectin. The other reason beans have a low glycemic index is because they are rich in fiber.

Fiber is a type of carbohydrate your body cannot absorb. In addition to beans, fiber can be found in vegetables, fruit (but not fruit juice), whole grains, seeds, and nuts. Eating fiber does not negate bad eating, but it can help in weight management by delaying the absorption of other carbohydrates you eat, and by keeping you full.

There are two types of fiber—soluble and insoluble. Soluble fiber dissolves in water and insoluble fiber does not. When soluble fiber is eaten with other foods, it forms a viscous gel complex that slows absorption, and results in a lowering of the glycemic index of the meal. Insoluble fiber passes through your gastrointestinal tract relatively intact, speeding up the passage of food through your intestine. This helps to relieve constipation, but it also makes you feel full sooner by triggering satiety hormones in your intestine.

These properties are the likely reasons why fiber consumption is effective for weight management. For instance, obesity is rare in populations that consume a high-fiber diet, and prevalent in populations that consume a low-fiber diet. Multiple studies have shown that fiber intake is inversely associated with weight gain.

And while fiber is important for weight management, it comes with some caveats. Fiber does not negate bad eating, and it certainly doesn't subtract bad carbohydrates from your system. Fiber is like sunscreen. Even if you apply sunscreen, you still want to protect yourself from toxic overexposure to the sun to prevent skin cancer. Likewise, chasing cookies and crackers with a fiber supplement doesn't erase the damaging effects of those refined processed snacks.

Furthermore, when soluble fiber is significantly processed, it loses its beneficial properties. This is why processed bread made from commercially milled flour still has a high glycemic index no matter how many grams of fiber it contains. Processed fiber doesn't make you feel as full as fiber eaten in its natural, whole form. One study found that people ate more after an appetizer of applesauce than they did after an appetizer of whole apples. This is why eating your fruits and vegetables is preferable to drinking them in the form of a juice or smoothie.

How much fiber is enough? I don't count calories and I don't count grams of carbohydrates, so do you think I count grams of fiber? Instead of counting the grams of fiber you eat over the course of your day, count on eating fruits, nonstarchy vegetables, beans, nuts, and seeds in the meals you eat every day. For instance, instead of cookies and cakes, reach for whole, unpeeled fruit. Instead of bread and rice, fill your bowl with beans. Instead of potato chips, have a handful of nuts. And of course…eat your vegetables. Let's talk about that next.

Chapter 20: E-at Your Vegetables!

"If it came from a plant, eat it; if it was made in a plant, don't."[13]

–Michael Pollan

Eat your vegetables. It seems like such simple advice. Most of us grew up hearing this from our mothers, and after all, mothers know best. Yet the typical American diet is sadly lacking in vegetables. In fact, one-third of all vegetables consumed in the United States come from just three pathetic sources: french fries, potato chips, and iceberg lettuce.

Why is our vegetable consumption so sad? Michael Pollan, an expert on the food industry and healthy eating gives us the answer. Pollan implicates our industrial food system for churning out an overabundance of cheap, processed food that has supplanted fresh, real food. So what's the solution? Taking into account all his prolific writing and meticulous research, Pollan summarizes his dietary advice with these few words: "Eat food. Not too much. Mostly plants."[14]

I used to think a vegetarian was someone who ate nothing but vegetables, and was therefore invariably healthy. To the contrary, I have worked with vegetarians who struggle mightily with their weight, because their diets consist of significant amounts of bad carbohydrates like processed grains. Instead of becoming a vegetarian, I ask you to become a vegetable-tarian.

If you have been doing the Ping Pong Diet, you have discovered firsthand the power of eating vegetables. The PP Diet is not just a low carbohydrate diet. It is designed to both keep you from eating bad carbohydrates, and turn you onto the power of plants and protein. I hope that your positive experience with the Ping Pong Diet has inspired you to become a vegetable-tarian. If I converted you, then I have done my job. In fact, the single most impactful dietary habit you can adopt for long-term weight management and health is to eat your vegetables.

Nonstarchy vegetables are packed with essential vitamins and minerals, high in fiber, and low in fat and glycemic index. Vegetables nourish your body and control your hunger, leaving less room in your stomach for fattening foods. In short, vegetables fill you up without filling you out. For example, in one study, subjects were given unlimited access to a main entree consisting of pasta and vegetables. The proportion of vegetables in the pasta dish was manipulated so that some people had pasta with a lot of vegetables, while other people had pasta with a small amount of vegetables. Regardless of which pasta dish people ate, they ended up eating the same amount of food by weight. As a result, people who ate the pasta dish with a lot of vegetables took in significantly fewer calories than people who ate the pasta dish with a small amount of vegetables.

In another study, obese women were counseled about weight management according to one of two strategies. Group A participants were given guidelines to reduce their fat intake. Group B participants were given the same guidelines to reduce their fat intake, but also instructed to incorporate satisfying amounts of fruits and vegetables into their diet. Despite reporting a similar reduction in total calories at six months, group B reported less hunger and had lost 33 percent more weight than group A.

You may have once been a victim of the processed food industry. You may have once fallen into a habit of eating take-out or fast food because it was convenient to do so. But that was in the past.

Instead of choosing processed fast food because it is convenient, make it convenient to eat fresh vegetables. Shop in grocery stores that stock fresh vegetables, instead of mini-marts that only stock processed foods. Stick to the periphery of the grocery store, where fresh produce is on display. In the wintertime, eat frozen vegetables that are picked and frozen at peak freshness. In the springtime, plant a vegetable garden, and check out your local farmers market. Consider joining a local nonprofit, community-supported agricultural co-op and get a weekly supply of fresh vegetables delivered to your door. In short, be a vegetable-tarian!

Chapter 21: E-xercise

When I counsel my patients on how to effectively lose weight, they are often perplexed that I focus primarily on diet and leave exercise out of the equation. You might find that puzzling, too. After all, I started this book by professing my love for the sport of ping pong, and throughout I've encouraged you to think like an elite athlete. Why haven't I suggested that you just play a vigorous game of ping pong to lose weight? Because it doesn't work!

An analysis of twenty-five years of weight loss research found that the average weight loss from aerobic exercise is only a little over six pounds.[15] Why is exercise so ineffective for weight loss? The answer lies in understanding what happens to your body both *during* and *after* exercise.

Let's take a hypothetical example of a 200-pound female named Mary, who decides to do some stationary rowing to lose weight. An hour of stationary rowing burns about 500 calories. There are approximately 3,500 calories in a pound of body fat. Therefore, if Mary rowed one hour daily, in one week she could theoretically lose one pound of fat. In six months, she could theoretically lose twenty-four pounds. However, this is deceivingly inaccurate, because the fuel you burn during exercise is not all fat.

Most people think they use short-term energy supplies like carbohydrates during light exercise, and tap into their fat at higher intensities. Surprisingly, studies show the opposite is true. Somewhat counterintuitively, during light exercise your body primarily burns fat as its source of energy (although, because it is low intensity, you don't burn through much fuel). However, as exercise intensity increases, your body increasingly uses carbohydrate sources such as glycogen stores for energy. During moderate intensity exercise, about half the fuel you use comes from carbohydrate sources and about half comes from your fat.

So, if Mary does a moderate intensity exercise like stationary rowing, only about half of the calories she burns would actually come from her fat stores. Therefore, it would take Mary closer to two weeks to burn off one pound of fat through exercise. This translates into rowing one hour daily for six months to burn off twelve pounds of fat.

However, even that is an overestimate of actual weight loss. This is due to compensation that occurs during the period immediately following exercise. Your body is a dynamic machine, constantly reacting to stimuli to maintain a steady and balanced state. After a period of exercise, your body senses that energy has been used, so it is primed to seek out and bring that energy back into your body. Let's explore this a little further.

First, although there is evidence that exercise causes an acute drop in appetite initially, about one hour post-exercise, your hormones actually increase your appetite. Second, studies show that people crave carbohydrates and eat more after a period of exercise. Third, once you do eat after you complete your exercise routine, your body has a tendency to more rapidly absorb the sugars in your meal, thus stimulating sharper insulin spikes and more fat storage. The net effect is that, post-exercise, energy is directed to flow back into your fat cells, once again fattening them up, and undoing a lot of the fat burning that took place during exercise.

The above compensatory mechanisms do not fully negate the amount of energy you expended during exercise, but they play a significant role in bringing energy back into your system, then storing that energy as fat. If, for instance, compensation were 50 percent effective, then Mary would ultimately lose only six pounds in six months by rowing one hour daily. This degree of weight loss is consistent with what is reported in studies.

You can't undo bad eating with exercise! And while exercise is an ineffective strategy for weight loss, it is an essential strategy to help you win at weight maintenance. Studies consistently show that active people are less likely to gain weight, and higher activity levels are predictive of successful long-term weight loss maintenance.

Exercise works for weight maintenance, but not in the way you might think. You might think that exercise affects weight by subtracting energy from your system, like taking a withdrawal out of your bank account. But I just explained that exercise is an inefficient means of burning fat. A better way of thinking about how exercise can be used for weight maintenance is to think about how exercise affects the *supply* of energy.

One study found that walking right after a meal is more effective for weight loss than walking one hour after eating. By the same token, exercising after your meals can help with your weight maintenance. Blood sugar levels increase and insulin levels spike after you eat a meal with carbohydrates. If you exercise soon after a meal, some of that meal's energy is used up, leading to lower blood sugar levels, lower insulin spikes, and less fat cell fattening. If calories eaten is analogous to income deposited into your body, exercise acts like an income tax, reducing the amount of leftover calories that can be stored as fat. Exercise also improves the action of insulin on muscle tissue, which helps divert energy to be burned by your muscles, rather than stored in your fat cells.

How much and what kind of exercise should you do? I recommend going for a sixty-minute brisk walk every day. A briskly paced walk is a pace of about 3.3 miles per hour, which is between a leisurely walk and a jog. Multiple studies show that moderate intensity exercise like a brisk walk is the optimum level of intensity for weight maintenance.

But the best thing about a brisk walk is anyone can do it. You don't have to be a trained athlete or have a personal trainer to go for a walk. It doesn't cost anything to go for a walk. You don't need any fancy gym equipment or a gym membership to go for a walk. Instead of carrying a change of clothes and squeezing in a trip to the gym before or after work, just go for a walk on your lunch break. Instead of plopping down in front of the television set after dinner, gather up your family and go for a walk.

If you make regular walking part of your lifestyle, exercise won't feel like a painful, time-consuming process. The key is to stop thinking of exercise as an isolated activity you *add* to your life, but rather an integral part of a healthy and active *way* of life. In the end, being more physically active will provide as much psychological benefit as physical benefit. Exercise is a great way to reflect the positive internal feelings and attitudes associated with being at a healthy weight. Thanks for reading. Now go for a walk!

Chapter 22: L-ean Protein Means Lean You

Everyone wants a lean, muscular body. What if I told you that you could build muscle without ever stepping foot in a gym? How do you do that? Eat protein. The Ping Pong Diet has already shown you the power of lean protein for weight loss. Eating lean protein is also a winning strategy for weight maintenance.

For example, in one study, people who lost 7.5 percent of their initial body weight were then followed for six months of weight maintenance. During maintenance, group A drank a daily thirty-gram protein drink, while group B had no additional supplement. At the end of six months, overall fat and belly fat decreased in group A, but increased in group B.[16] Also, not only did group A regain less weight at a slower rate than group B, but the mass gained by group A was entirely muscle mass!

How does eating protein help prevent fattening? Incorporating protein into your meals lowers the glycemic index and keeps you full. In addition, eating protein uses up energy and increases your metabolism. When I was a boy, I used to complain that eating made me tired. It turns out that I wasn't *just* being a whiny little kid. Eating actually does use up energy. You burn up a small amount of energy to digest, absorb, and dispose of the food you eat, which is called the thermic effect of food. The thermic effect of eating protein is significantly greater than that of eating carbohydrates or fat.

Eating protein also increases your metabolism. In one study, after achieving a weight loss of 13.6 percent of their initial body weight over twelve weeks, participants were then randomized to weight maintenance diets that varied in protein content. At the end of four weeks, subjects who were maintained on a diet consisting of 30 percent protein had significantly higher metabolisms than subjects who were maintained on a diet consisting of 20 percent protein.[17]

It turns out that your metabolism is highly correlated with the amount of muscle mass you have. Essentially, the more muscle you have, the more energy you use for day-to-day functioning because muscle is a metabolically active organ. You may not have realized it, but before you started the Ping Pong Diet, the number on your scale reflected *both* higher fat *and* higher muscle mass! With weight loss, you lose both fat and muscle mass, and as you lose muscle, your metabolism slows. This is why the rate of weight loss often slows down with prolonged dieting. You may have experienced this roadblock in your own weight loss efforts. What's worse, the slowing in metabolism that occurs with weight loss sets you up to regain weight. So what can you do? Eat protein! By keeping protein intake high during weight loss and weight maintenance, you can rebuild metabolically active muscle mass, and offset some of the slowing in your metabolism.

But make sure to continue eating lean sources of protein like you have been doing on the Ping Pong Diet. By eating lean protein, you can actually build lean muscle mass without ever stepping foot in a gym. Therefore, lean protein means lean you. Literally.

Chapter 23: W-hole or Not at All

The other day, I baked a batch of cookies using whole oats, nuts, and peanut butter. I took a large cookie, broke it in half, and gave it to my son Colin. That was a mistake. His face turned red, his upper lip thinned, and his eyes began to well up. "The WHOLE thing! I want the WHOLE thing!" he cried.

When it comes to grains, you too should be up in arms. You, too, should demand the whole thing! I already declared processed bread as being the most flagrant example of sugar in disguise. In the case of processed bread, the original wheat berry grain is pulverized into fine flour that is rapidly absorbed when eaten. In some cases, the fibrous layer of the wheat berry grain is removed during processing. In other cases, the fiber is not removed, but it is so decimated by the milling process that it loses any beneficial properties. In either case, the result is processed bread with a high glycemic index.

Don't bother looking for processed products made out of whole grains. Just eat actual whole grains. I say, "Eat it whole or not at all." Whole grains contain all the original layers of the grain, including the starchy endosperm, the germ layer (high in vitamin B complexes and magnesium), and the outer bran layer (high in fiber). By eating grains in their whole form, you not only get important vitamins and minerals, you also get the full benefit of eating unprocessed fiber.

Examples of whole grains include oats, quinoa, farro, bulgur, barley, popcorn, wheat berries, rye berries, spelt, amaranth, buckwheat, and kasha. If you go to a grocery store looking for some quinoa, the ingredient list on the box should say...quinoa! That's it. Just quinoa.

Study after study demonstrate a strong inverse association between whole grain consumption and risk of diabetes, heart disease, and weight gain.[18] For instance, one study found that belly fat was 10 percent lower in individuals consuming three or more servings of whole grains per day compared with those who essentially consumed no whole grains.[19] An important finding in this study was that the positive effects of eating whole grains only occurred when highly processed, refined grains were *replaced* by whole grains. The positive effects of whole grain consumption were nullified when whole grains were just simply *added* to continued consumption of refined grains.

This last finding is an important distinction, and is the basis for why I recommend eating it whole or not at all. The other day I came across the latest dietary guidelines from the US Department of Agriculture. I was bewildered by their recommendations for eating grains. Instead of recommending Americans replace all refined grains with whole grains, the guidelines stated, "At least half of recommended total grain intake should be whole grains."

This is entirely missing the point. Because grains are dense in carbohydrates, higher in glycemic index, and make up a large portion of the American diet, they play a prominent role in our country's struggle with obesity. The emphasis should not be to incorporate a minimum amount of whole grains in your diet, but to avoid excessive intake of grains, and eliminate refined grains altogether. In other words, "Eat it whole or not at all!"

Instead of the obligatory sandwich for lunch, sprinkle whole grains onto salads and other vegetables. Try whole bulgur in a delicious tabouleh salad with fresh tomatoes and cucumbers. Instead of potato chips, snack on some air-popped popcorn. Rather than pour yourself a bowl of processed cereal, why not cook up some warm quinoa and top it with fruit? Or, bake up a batch of cookies using whole oats, nuts, and peanut butter. Just make sure you share the WHOLE thing.

Chapter 24: E-ating System for Transition and Maintenance

As you approach your goal weight, you will need to prepare yourself for the transition from the Ping Pong Diet to an eating system that balances fat burning and fat storage. The Ping Pong Diet is designed to be so simple to implement, it becomes habit. As you approach the time to transition off the Ping Pong Diet, it is normal to feel somewhat anxious. Don't worry! The habits you have already developed by following the Ping Pong Diet, and the strategies you have learned throughout the twenty-one point plan for weight maintenance, have prepared you for this transition.

The purpose of transitioning is to acclimate your body to the carbohydrates restricted during weight loss, while minimizing weight regain. As in the Ping Pong Diet, plants and protein will remain the foundation of your eating system during transition and maintenance. Protein sources will continue to be low in saturated fat. Likewise, you will continue to control your hunger by eating five times a day, in a portion- and proportion-controlled way, as you transition from eating five meals a day to eating three meals and two snacks a day.

Whereas restriction of carbohydrate quantity was the main focus of the Ping Pong Diet, attention to carbohydrate quality through low glycemic eating will be your primary focus during transition and into maintenance. You will reintroduce different categories of carbohydrates one at a time, according to increasing glycemic index. You will also continue to limit the highest glycemic index foods like sugars, sugary beverages, starchy root vegetables, bread, and rice.

Here is an overview of your transition from the Ping Pong Diet to maintenance:

Transition:

Week 1: Continue Ping Pong Diet, but you may incorporate onions, brussels sprouts, artichokes, and okra.

	Additional Carbs	Quantity	Meals	Snacks
Week 2:	Nuts	Handful	5	0
Week 3:	Nonfat Dairy	1 cup/day	4	1
Week 4:	Legumes	1 cup/day	4	1
Week 5:	Fruit	1 cup/day	3	2
Week 6:	Whole Grains	1/2 cup/day	3	2

Transitioning typically takes place over six weeks. However, if you have lost more than fifty pounds on the Ping Pong Diet, you should consider spreading your transition out over twelve weeks. The transition is organized in a logical stepwise sequence based on incremental increases in glycemic index. This is designed to make you think about categories of carbohydrates based on weight gain potential. Also, because a foundation of nonstarchy vegetables and lean protein is all your body needs nutritionally, additional carbohydrates can be lumped together conceptually as icing on the cake.

Each week, add back one of the categories, and continue to monitor your weight on a weekly basis. Monitoring your weight will help you evaluate how your body responds to specific carbohydrates. If you notice that a specific category of carbohydrates is associated with weight gain for you, pull back on the quantity of that carbohydrate grouping, and substitute with carbohydrates that do not cause weight gain for you. Be aware that carbohydrates with higher glycemic indices have greater potential for weight gain, so be especially careful when adding back whole grains.

During week one of your transition, you will continue the structured eating system of the Ping Pong Diet, but you can now eat onions, brussels sprouts, artichokes, and okra. These vegetables were excluded during the weight loss phase due to higher carbohydrate content, but are allowed during transition and maintenance because they are low in glycemic index. Starchy root vegetables that are high in glycemic index (potatoes, sweet potatoes, yams, taro, beets, turnips, parsnip, carrots, winter squash, pumpkin, peas, and corn) are still excluded.

In week two of your transition, you will add a handful of nuts per day to the standard five meals of the Ping Pong Diet. In week three, you will drop one of the meals of the Ping Pong Diet, and add one cup of nonfat plain Greek yogurt per day to the handful of nuts, which will serve as a snack. By week four, you will add one cup of beans per day, which can be spread out over your four meals. I recommend you start with edamame or black beans you cook yourself (not canned), because they are lower in glycemic index.

By week five of your transition, you will drop another of the meals from the Ping Pong Diet and add one cup of fruit. Fruit topped with some nuts for added protein serves as your second daily snack.

I recommend you choose low glycemic fruit like blackberries or raspberries, and avoid high glycemic fruit like bananas and melons. In week six, you can add one-half cup of whole grains to one of your three meals.

At the completion of your transition, your maintenance eating system will consist of three meals and two snacks per day. Meals will consist of two cups of nonstarchy vegetables, one lean protein the size of a deck of cards, and one-half cup of either beans or whole grains. Your two snacks will consist of one cup of yogurt and one cup of fruit along with a handful of nuts divided between the two. The order of your meals and snacks doesn't matter, as long as you are eating approximately every three hours. For instance, you might choose to eat a meal at 8:00 a.m., 2:00 p.m., and 8:00 p.m., and have your snacks in between meals at 11:00 a.m. and 5:00 p.m. Alternatively, you might choose to start and end your day with a snack and have three meals in between.

If your weight fluctuates, you need to adjust your proportions accordingly. If you find yourself gaining weight, you may need to increase your intake of lean protein and nonstarchy plants, and back off on the other sources of carbohydrates. Likewise, if you find yourself losing weight, you may need to increase the proportions of your other carbohydrates.

Remember that sugars, sugary beverages, bread, rice, and starchy root vegetables are high in glycemic index and particularly fattening. You should be very cautious with these foods, and eat these foods sparingly, if at all. If you do choose to eat bread or rice, consider lower glycemic options such as sourdough, sprouted grain bread, and long grain rice, like basmati rice.

Just as the Ping Pong Diet was foreign at first, this eating system for transition and maintenance will feel unusual initially. When I played competitive ping pong, I went through countless changes in my forehand. Although awkward at first, with practice, I developed a better forehand. You've been eating a certain way your entire life. Changing what you eat, and the way you eat, is bound to be awkward at first. But with repetition, eating in this new way will begin feeling less unnatural and more like second nature. Your expectations will change. Your taste buds will change. Your habits will change. You will go from dieting to dominating.

Chapter 25: L-earn to Manage Your Mind

Run one mile under four minutes. There was a time when achieving this feat was thought to be physically impossible and mentally unfathomable. Why? Because no one had done it before. In *The Perfect Mile*[20], Neal Bascomb tells the story of Roger Bannister, John Landy, and Wes Santee, three world-class runners who each set out to break the four-minute mile in the early 1950s. He tracks the intense training regimen and singular focus of each of these men, who, despite being on three different continents, were able to push one another closer and closer to reaching that elusive goal. And then in 1954, the Englishman Bannister broke the barrier with a time of 3:59.4.

Competitive running is one of the best examples of awe-inspiring human potential on display. Equal parts physical strength and mental toughness, running is as much a competition with others as it is with yourself. Competition can either wear you down, or it can push you to achieve something seemingly impossible.

In many ways, managing your weight is like being an elite runner. Perhaps your goal weight is *your* four-minute mile. Some days you may feel like managing your weight is a walk in the park. Some days you may even hit such a stride with your weight management that it feels like a runner's high. Other days you may feel emotionally and physically exhausted, as if you can't take another step. And just as the guy running in the lane next to you can serve as both motivation and competition, your mind can be your friend or your foe. Your mind can tell you to procrastinate, and even to abdicate. Your mind can also tell you to dominate.

In *THINK*, Dr. Stewart Zelman references the saying, "The mind is a great slave and a terrible master." You can let negative thoughts control and define you, or you can manage your mind to master yourself and determine who you want to be. Your friends don't define you. Your coworkers don't define you. Society doesn't define you. Only *you* define you. Whether or not you decide to become the master of your own mind is entirely up to you. In fact, the only person you have complete and total control over is you.

Taking control of your mind begins with changing negative thought patterns. When your mind tells you that your weight management can wait, that you're too tired to stick to your plan, or that processed junk food doesn't really harm your health, change your mind! Dr. Zelman teaches people to manage their minds by changing the language they use to speak to themselves. Use the present or future tense to refer to any behavior that is positive or desirable. Alternatively, use the past tense to refer to undesirable behaviors. Instead of saying, "I always eat a cookie after dinner," say, "I used to always eat a cookie after dinner. That doesn't define who I am anymore."

Sometimes your mind can be a bully. Like the big kid on the playground, your mind may attack your confidence, or tell you that you can't do something. You may have struggled with food and your weight all your life. It is only natural to have occasional feelings of helplessness. Again, it comes down to human potential. We all have the potential to be great. You may not have always been great when it comes to healthy food choices, but you are great at something. You may be an excellent piano player, or a trivia whiz. In my case, ping pong is how I once distinguished myself.

One successful technique Dr. Zelman practices is to have people picture themselves doing something they are masterful at, then transfer those associated feelings of control and confidence into a mental image of themselves doing something they have struggled with. This exercise helps people learn that, just as they can be masterful at one thing, they can manage their mind to master their body weight.

Although all good runners have physical skill, championship runners have championship mentality. Having a championship mentality can help you get to your four-minute mile. But even more important than reaching the goals you set for yourself is carrying that championship mentality forward through weight maintenance and beyond. Once you learn to master your mind, not only will you reach the finish line, there will be no looking back.

Chapter 26: L-ive!

Perhaps at one point or another during this book you said to yourself, "I can't eat this. I can't eat that. That's no way to live!" You enjoy food. I enjoy food. What human being doesn't enjoy food? It's in our nature. It's one of the great pleasures of life. When I started practicing weight management, I was so busy trying to prescribe the right thing for my patients that I nearly forgot how hard it is to ask someone to give up the wrong things. I quickly learned that asking anyone to give up anything, right or wrong, is asking that individual to feel deprived in some way.

I agree that living a deprived life is no way to live. Being deprived of the knowledge of where your food comes from is no way to live. Being deprived of the knowledge of how much added sugars are in your food is no way to live. Eating nutritionally poor, processed food, and being deprived of true nourishment is no way to live. Eating a high glycemic diet and developing otherwise preventable diseases like diabetes and heart disease is no way to live. You see, choosing to eat processed foods that deprive you of your vitality IS choosing the path of deprivation. Choosing to eliminate harmful foods from your diet is choosing to *live*!

As a doctor, I am tasked with the preservation of life. Like most internists, I have seen patients through infections, neurological disease, heart failure, and even cancer. But the only time a grown man has been so moved as to give me a bear hug is after I helped him to lose, and keep off, significant weight. In fact, helping my patients lose weight, maintain weight loss, and get back to a healthy existence has been one of the most gratifying aspects of my professional career. Despite being called a health provider, before practicing bariatric medicine, I was more in the business of controlling unhealthiness, than in the business of providing healthiness. Using food to create health has allowed me to care for my patients in a way no medication has ever allowed me to do.

Practicing bariatric medicine has given me the opportunity to witness remarkable transformations. People who had taken two, three, or four medications for diabetes, high blood pressure, and elevated cholesterol are able to stop taking medications altogether. They feel more energetic and confident. They are able to do more, and live more active lifestyles. People who lose weight simply *feel* better.

And while the process of losing weight feels great, and is typically accompanied by kind remarks from family and friends, weight maintenance is the true reward. True success stems from taking pride in your body and your health. Health is both the final solution and the ultimate reward. That's why the ultimate goal isn't defined by a number, but by achieving and internalizing values of lifelong health. When health becomes a value that defines who you are as a person, you will undoubtedly win at weight maintenance.

Winning at weight maintenance does not come with a medal or a plaque. Instead, you can look at yourself in the mirror and take pride in the knowledge of what you have been able to accomplish. You beat genetics. You beat your toxic food environment. You took control over your mind and body. You did what 80 percent of dieters fail to do. You maintained your weight! You can take pride in continually achieving one of the hardest things one can do—a lifetime achievement award, if you will. You are winning at weight maintenance. You are living life to the fullest. Now *that* is how you *live*!

Ping Pong Diet Recipes

Thai Chicken with Roasted Broccoli

Serving size: 5 meals per recipe

Ingredients
- 1-1/2 lb. chicken breast
- 2 tablespoons fish sauce
- 1 tablespoon curry powder
- 1/2 teaspoons black pepper
- 2 tablespoons canola oil
- 20 cups broccoli, trimmed
- 1-1/2 teaspoons salt
- 1 teaspoon red pepper flakes

Directions
1. Trim excess fat from chicken.
2. Marinate chicken in fish sauce, curry powder, black pepper, and 1/2 teaspoon oil overnight.
3. Grill chicken till cooked through.
4. Preheat oven to 400 degrees Fahrenheit.
5. Mix broccoli with 1-1/2 tablespoons canola oil, salt, and red pepper flakes.
6. Roast broccoli for 30 minutes.
7. Serve chicken with broccoli and enjoy.

Steak and Tomatoes

Serving size: 5 meals per recipe

Ingredients
- 1-1/2 lb. beef eye of round roast
- Salt and pepper to taste
- 20 cups grape tomatoes, halved
- 2 tablespoons canola oil
- 4 tablespoons balsamic vinegar
- 1 cup fresh basil, torn

Directions
1. Preheat oven to 500 degrees Fahrenheit.
2. Trim excess fat from beef.
3. Season beef with salt and pepper, place in a roasting pan in oven, and roast for 8 minutes.
4. Turn off oven, but do not open for two hours.
5. Mix 20 cups grape tomatoes with oil, vinegar, and basil, and serve with thin slices of roast beef.

Lemon Chicken with Summer Squash

Serving size: 5 meals per recipe

Ingredients
- 1-1/2 lbs. chicken breast
- 1 tablespoon lemon zest
- 1 tablespoon chopped fresh thyme
- 1/4 teaspoon salt
- 1/4 teaspoon freshly ground black pepper
- 10 cups zucchini
- 10 cups yellow summer squash
- 1/4 cup chicken broth

Directions
1. Trim fat from chicken.
2. Toss lemon zest and thyme and split into two bowls.
3. Add 1/4 teaspoon salt and 1/4 teaspoon black pepper to one of the lemon-thyme mixtures, then sprinkle on chicken.
4. Heat 1/2 tablespoon canola oil in a nonstick skillet over medium-high heat.
5. Cook chicken until golden on both sides, and cooked through.
6. Cut squash into 1/2-inch pieces.
7. Sauté squash in nonstick skillet over medium heat, stirring frequently, until golden and tender. Stir in remaining lemon-thyme mixture and chicken broth.
8. Serve chicken with squash and enjoy.

Spice Rubbed Pork with Napa Cabbage

Serving size: 5 meals per recipe

Ingredients
- 1-1/2 lb. pork tenderloin
- Sugar-free dry rub (i.e., McCormick Grill Mates Chipotle & Roasted Garlic)
- 2 tablespoons canola oil
- 20 cups napa cabbage
- 4 cloves garlic
- 1/4 cup chicken broth

Directions
1. Preheat oven to 450 degrees Fahrenheit.
2. Trim fat from pork.
3. Rub spice mixture on pork until thickly coated on all sides.
4. Cover and refrigerate overnight.
5. Heat 1 tablespoon canola oil in a 10- to 12-in. heavy frying pan over medium-high heat.
6. Pan sear pork 1–2 minutes per side.
7. Transfer pork to roasting pan and bake for 20 minutes.
8. Brown garlic in frying pan on high heat.
9. Add chicken broth and napa cabbage, bring to a boil, cover, and cook until tender.
10. Serve napa cabbage with sliced pork.

Steamed Fish with Bok Choy

Serving size: 5 meals per recipe

Ingredients
- 1-1/2 lbs. whole red snapper
- 2 tablespoons canola oil
- 1/4 cup soy sauce
- 1 tablespoon rice wine
- 2 inches ginger, peeled and julienned
- 5 sprigs cilantro
- 20 cups bok choy, chopped
- 1/4 cup chicken broth
- 2 garlic cloves, minced
- Salt and pepper to taste

Directions
1. Rinse fish, then season with salt and pepper.
2. Stuff fish with ginger.
3. Fill bottom of steamer with one inch water and bring to a boil.
4. Place fish on steamer rack and steam for 8 minutes, until flaky.
5. Lay sprigs of cilantro on top of fish.
6. Heat oil, then pour over fish.
7. Mix soy sauce and rice wine and pour over fish.
8. Brown garlic in frying pan over high heat, add chicken broth and bok choy, bring to a boil, then cover and cook until tender.
9. Serve chunks of fish with bok choy.

Bloody Mary Salmon with Roasted Cauliflower

Serving size: 5 meals per recipe

Ingredients
- 1-1/2 lbs. salmon fillets
- 1-1/2 cups bloody mary mix
- 20 cups cauliflower, trimmed
- 1-1/2 teaspoons salt
- 1 teaspoon red pepper flakes
- Black pepper to taste

Directions
1. Preheat oven to 400 degrees Fahrenheit.
2. Place salmon fillets in a medium baking dish and season with salt and pepper.
3. Pour bloody mary mix over fillets, cover, and refrigerate for 30 minutes.
4. Preheat broiler on high.
5. Broil salmon for 7 minutes, until fish is flaky.
6. Mix cauliflower with oil, salt, red pepper flakes, and black pepper.
7. Roast cauliflower for 30 minutes.
8. Serve salmon with cauliflower and enjoy.

Mustard Roasted Salmon and Asparagus

Serving size: 5 meals per recipe

Ingredients
- 1-1/2 lbs. salmon fillets
- 2 tablespoons rice wine vinegar
- 4 tablespoons stone-ground mustard
- 1 garlic clove, minced
- 1 tablespoon parsley, chopped
- 1 tablespoon chives, chopped
- 1/2 tablespoon thyme, chopped
- 20 cups asparagus, ends removed
- 1-1/2 tablespoons canola oil
- 1-1/2 teaspoons salt
- 1 teaspoon red pepper flakes
- Black pepper to taste

Directions
1. Preheat oven to 400 degrees Fahrenheit.
2. In a small bowl, combine vinegar, mustard, garlic, and herbs.
3. Place salmon pieces on a sheet pan lined with parchment paper. Season with salt and pepper. Brush mustard glaze onto salmon.
4. Bake for 15 minutes, until flaky.
5. Mix asparagus with oil, salt, red pepper flakes, and black pepper.
6. Roast asparagus for 30 minutes.
7. Serve salmon with asparagus and enjoy.

Kale Salad with Eggplant and Rotisserie Chicken

Ingredients

- 18 cups kale
- 1 teaspoon salt
- 2 tablespoons canola oil
- 1 cup eggplant, cooked
- 1 garlic clove, minced
- 1/2 lemon, juiced
- 1 rotisserie chicken

Directions

1. Preheat oven to 400 degrees Fahrenheit.
2. Chop kale and remove stems.
3. Massage kale with 1 tablespoon of canola oil and 1 teaspoon salt.
4. Roast 1 small eggplant in oven for 40 minutes.
5. Cool eggplant and peel.
6. Place eggplant, garlic, 1 tablespoon oil, and lemon juice in food processor, and puree until smooth.
7. Remove skin from rotisserie chicken, and tear chicken into strips.
8. Mix kale, eggplant dressing, and chicken strips and serve.

Deconstructed Shrimp Sushi

Serving size: 5 meals per recipe

Ingredients
- 1 pound frozen cooked, peeled shrimp
- 20 cups kale, stems removed
- 2 tablespoons canola oil
- 1 tablespoon sesame oil
- 3 tablespoons rice vinegar
- 2 tablespoons soy sauce
- 2 garlic cloves
- 1/8 teaspoon red pepper flakes
- 1 teaspoon salt
- Soy sauce and wasabi paste to taste, for dipping

Directions
1. Thaw shrimp in refrigerator overnight.
2. Remove tails and peel shrimp.
3. Chop kale and remove stems.
4. Dress kale in oil, vinegar, soy sauce, cloves, red pepper flakes, and salt.
5. Serve shrimp atop kale salad with soy sauce and wasabi for dipping.

Tuna Salad with Miso Ginger Dressing

Serving size: 5 meals per recipe

Ingredients
- 4 five-ounce cans of tuna in vegetable oil
- 20 cups romaine lettuce
- 1 tablespoon sesame oil
- 3 tablespoons rice vinegar
- 2 tablespoons soy sauce
- 1 tablespoon minced ginger
- 1 tablespoon miso paste

Directions
1. Chop lettuce and dress with oil, vinegar, soy sauce, ginger, and miso paste.
2. Top with tuna and serve.

References

1. A. Thorogood, et al., "Isolated Aerobic Exercise and Weight Loss: A Systematic Review and Meta-analysis of Randomized Controlled Trials," *American Journal of Medicine* 124(8) (August 2011):747-55.

2. Foster, et al., "A Randomized Trial of a Low Carbohydrate Diet for Obesity," *New England Journal of Medicine* 348(21) (2003):2082-2090.

3. Samaha, et al. "A Low Carbohydrate, as Compared with a Low Fat Diet in Severe Obesity," *New England Journal of Medicine* 348(21) (2003):2074-2081.

4. N. Santesso, et al., "Effects of Higher Versus Lower Protein Diets on Health Outcomes: A Systematic Review and Meta-analysis," *European Journal of Clinical Nutrition* 66 (2012):780-788.

5. D.K. Layman, et al., "A Reduced Ratio of Dietary Carbohydrate to Protein Improves Body Composition and Blood Lipid Profiles During Weight Loss in Adult Women," *Journal of Nutrition* 133 (2003):411-417.

6. Malcolm Gladwell, *Outliers: The Story of Success* (New York: Little, Brown and Co., 2008).

7. Charles Duhigg, *The Power of Habit: Why We Do What We Do in Life and Business* (New York: Random House, 2012).

8. Stuart A. Zelman, PhD, *THINK: Mindful and Mindless Tools for Weight Management* (Bloomington:Authorhouse, 2012).

9. S. Liu, et al., "Relation Between Changes in Intakes of Dietary Fiber and Grain Products and Changes in Weight and Development of Obesity Among Middle-aged Women," *American Journal of Clinical Nutrition* 78 (2003):920-7.

10. J. Salmeron, et al., "Dietary Fiber, Glycemic Load, and Risk of NIDDM in Men," *Diabetes Care* 20 (1997):545-50.

11. J.M. Shikany, et al., "Association of Glycemic Load with Cardiovascular Disease Risk Factors: The Women's Health Initiative Observational Study," *Nutrition* 26(6) (2010):641-647.

12. William Davis, 2011, *Wheat Belly: Lose the Wheat, Lose the Weight, and Find Your Path Back to Health* (New York: Rodale books, 2011).

13. Michael Pollan, *Food Rules: An Eater's Manual* (New York: Penguin Group, 2009).

14. Michael Pollan, *In Defense of Food: An Eater's Manifesto* (New York: Penguin Group, 2008).

15. T. Wu, et al., "Long-term Effectiveness of Diet-Plus-Exercise Interventions vs. Diet-Only Interventions for Weight Loss: A Meta-analysis," *Obesity Review* 10 (2009:313-323).

16. M.S. Westerterp-Plantenga, et al., "High Protein Intake Sustains Weight Maintenance After Body Weight Loss in Humans," *International Journal of Obesity Related Metabolic Disorders* 28(1) (January 2004:57-64).

17. T.M. Larsen, et al. "Diets with High or Low Protein Content and Glycemic Index for Weight Loss Maintenance," *New England Journal of Medicine* 363(22) (2010:2102-2113).

18. E.Q. Ye, et al., "Greater Whole Grain Intake is Associated with Lower Risk of Type 2 Diabetes, Cardiovascular Disease, and Weight Gain," *Journal of Nutrition* (2012).

19. N.M. McKeown, et al., "Whole and Refined Grain Intakes Are Differentially Associated with Abdominal Visceral and Subcutaneous Adiposity in Healthy Adults: The Framingham Heart Study," *American Journal of Clinical Nutrition* 92 (2010:1165-71).

20. Neal Bascomb, *The Perfect Mile: Three Athletes, One Goal, and Less Than Four Minutes to Achieve It* (Boston: Hougton Mifflin Co., 2004).

40678476R00085

Made in the USA
Middletown, DE
19 February 2017